"As a naturopathic physician with a general practice, I not infrequently encounter patients suffering from generalized anxiety and panic disorder. I have recommended Bourne's previous books for these patients, and they have found them rich resources for learning coping skills to ultimately overcome their worries and fears.

"This latest book is a clear overview of many of the effective strategies employed by naturopathic physicians and other holistic practitioners to address the multiple contributors to anxiety and its related disorders, including dietary factors, hypoglycemia, adrenal exhaustion, toxicity, premenstrual syndrome, and insufficient exercise.

"Following the dietary and lifestyle recommendations contained in this book will reliably lead to the fading away of anxiety and panic."

—Michael Traub, ND, past president of the American Association of Naturopathic Physicians and a naturopathic physician in private practice in Kailua Kona, HI and Marin County, CA

NATURAL
Relief for
ANXIETY

*Complementary
Strategies for
Easing Fear,
Panic & Worry*

EDMUND J. BOURNE, PH.D.
ARLEN BROWNSTEIN, ND
LORNA GARANO

New Harbinger Publications, Inc.

Publisher's Note

Distributed in Canada by Raincoast Books.

New Harbinger Publications, Inc.
5674 Shattuck Avenue
Oakland, CA 94609

Cover design by Amy Shoup
Text design by Michele Waters-Kermes
Acquired by Catharine Sutker
Edited by Jessica Beebe

ISBN 1-57224-372-4 Paperback

Printed in the United States of America

New Harbinger Publications' Web site address: www.newharbinger.com

06   05   04

10   9   8   7   6   5   4   3   2   1

First printing

Table of Contents

Introduction

Anxiety is an inevitable part of life for most of us. A majority of people report that they worry about issues such as finances, health, and family on a daily basis. A smaller number, about 15 percent of adults, have a diagnosable anxiety disorder such as panic attacks, agoraphobia (multiple phobias), social phobia, obsessive-compulsive disorder, or post-traumatic stress disorder. It's apparent that the stress of modern life—the pace, the complexity, the level of social alienation, and the lack of consensual standards to live by—takes its toll on many of us. Whether you are dealing with everyday worries and anxiety or have more intense and lasting anxiety symptoms in the form of a specific anxiety disorder, this book offers you a variety of strategies to help you achieve a calmer, more peaceful way of life.

Conventional help for anxiety and anxiety disorders can be found in numerous books. I've presented such an approach in *The Anxiety & Phobia Workbook* and *Coping with Anxiety,* and this kind of help can be found in scores of other good books. The conventional approach to overcoming anxiety difficulties combines *cognitive behavioral therapy* (CBT) with prescription medication. CBT typically includes relaxation therapy, replacing fearful what-if thinking with more realistic, supportive self-talk and beliefs, and gradually facing—in small increments—the situations you fear and avoid. Chapters 1 and 4 of this book cover some of the strategies used in CBT. Prescription medications, while quite helpful for more severe anxiety conditions, are not covered in this book.

This book takes a unique approach in emphasizing strictly natural methods for overcoming anxiety. Thus it will be most helpful for everyday anxiety, or for anxiety issues that are in the mild to moderate range. *Mild to moderate* means your problem with anxiety can be bothersome at times and causes you some distress on occasion or in specific situations. However, it does not disrupt your life in a major way, preventing you from working or maintaining satisfactory relationships, or causing you significant distress more than half of the time. *Mild to moderate* means you can cope with your anxiety but would like some additional help. More severe anxiety conditions generally overwhelm your coping resources and are best treated with a combination of cognitive behavioral therapy, the techniques included in this book, and medication. If, for example, you are dealing with daily panic attacks, severe social phobia (fear of being in any group situation), obsessions and compulsions, or post-traumatic stress disorder, you may well benefit from a course of medication in addition to the approaches described in this book. For an in-depth discussion of medication, please see the chapter on medication in *The Anxiety & Phobia Workbook*.

The natural approaches described here differ from mainstream cognitive behavioral therapy and medication in two ways. First, most of the methods (with the exception of relaxation, exercise, and the cognitive interventions in chapter 4) have not yet been validated by empirical research as treatment methods for anxiety. They have, however, proven helpful to large numbers of people dealing with anxiety as well as a variety of other conditions. This is evident from reports I've received from my own clients. Beyond this, thousands of holistic practitioners around the world have reported methods such as diet, herbs, meditation, yoga, massage, and acupuncture to be helpful in general. There is research supporting all of these modalities, just not specific studies examining their efficacy with anxiety in particular. My recommendation is that you give each of the methods described in this book a fair trial. Work with one method (or more) on a daily basis for one month, then evaluate how you feel that method has affected your condition. (For massage, acupuncture, or chiropractic, one session per week for a month would constitute a fair trial.)

Second, the approach taken in this book differs from mainstream approaches in that it is fundamentally holistic. It addresses the whole person. CBT primarily addresses only two components of the person: *cognitions* (assumptions and beliefs) and *acquired habits* developed through conditioning. Medication addresses only physiology or neurotransmitter imbalances in the brain. Rather than offering specific techniques that target your behavior or brain physiology, most of the strategies in this book address you as a whole person. As you read through the following chapters, you'll explore how

- changing your diet and using supplements may result in greater calmness throughout the day;

- dealing with conditions such as hypoglycemia, food allergies, adrenal exhaustion, candida, toxicity, PMS, and seasonal affective disorder can reduce anxiety and improve feelings of well-being;

- simplifying your life can help you achieve greater peace of mind;

- learning to meditate regularly can reduce worry and emotional reactivity;

- embracing a more spiritual outlook might offer a deep healing in your life.

Working with any of these methods will help your whole life to improve. Your problem with anxiety—whether everyday worry, panic, generalized anxiety, or phobias—will improve, and so may your depression, headaches, insomnia, mood swings, irritability, and so on. In short, *all* of you will get better.

Some of the material in this book has not been presented in any other self-help books on anxiety, to my knowledge. The health conditions we discuss in chapter 5 that can impact anxiety (adrenal exhaustion, candida, general toxicity, heavy metal toxicity, and seasonal affective disorder) are not described in any books on anxiety I've seen, yet it is equally important to address these conditions as it is more commonly known conditions such as hypoglycemia and food allergies. Several books have mentioned yoga as a very helpful intervention to promote relaxation and an inner balance that can reduce anxiety. I feel similar consideration should be given to tai chi and qi gong. Finally, the chapter on spirituality introduces a perspective that has been largely neglected in most self-help books on anxiety.

The ultimate basis for including some of these less well-known approaches is my personal experience. This experience includes both my own recovery from an anxiety disorder (a combination of OCD and panic disorder) and the recovery of many of my clients. Meditation, yoga, diet, detoxification, herbs, massage, chiropractic, and spirituality have been helpful to me personally and to many persons I've worked with. So I encourage you to try such methods. If you are already receiving cognitive behavioral therapy or medication for an anxiety disorder, consider these alternative methods as adjuncts to your treatment. I believe you won't be disappointed in the results.

This book can only provide the briefest introduction to most of the topics it covers. Many volumes have been written on diet, herbs, supplements, hypoglycemia, food allergies, detoxification, meditation, yoga, qi gong, how to simplify your life, and self-help spirituality. A brief list of suggestions for further reading, organized by topic, can be found at the end of this book.

I wish you the best in your efforts to overcome your difficulties with anxiety. I expect you'll find many of the natural approaches described in this book to be helpful. There is much help available, and I believe that a high level of recovery is always possible if you're sincerely committed to achieving it.

—Ed Bourne, Ph.D.

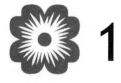 1

Relaxation

If you're like most people, you think that your ability to relax is like your ability to walk or sleep: a built-in mechanism that works without effort or training. This is why it's so easy to tell yourself to "just relax," and why you can get so frustrated when nothing happens in response. The truth is that to achieve real relaxation, it helps to master certain skills. In this way relaxation is closer to an active exercise like playing the piano than a passive one like sleeping. If you were taking piano lessons, you would have to commit to a certain amount of time for daily practice. The same is true for learning relaxation skills. By regularly practicing the relaxation exercises in this chapter, you'll reduce the occurrence of anxiety symptoms, and you'll gain essential skills for freeing yourself from them when they arise.

The Four Signs of Relaxation

How do you know when you are relaxed? There are four characteristic signs of relaxation:

1. You are able to breathe easily and deeply, filling both your chest cavity and abdominal area.

2. The muscles throughout your body feel soft, loose, flexible, and unconstrained.

3. Your heart beats calmly and regularly, easily circulating your blood throughout your body so that your hands and feet are usually warm.

4. Your mind is clear and calm; you are undistracted and can concentrate easily.

The Anatomy of Relaxation

When you are relaxed, a distinct part of your autonomic nervous system, the *parasympathetic nervous system,* is activated. The parasympathetic nervous system is responsible for maintaining normal function of your internal organ systems in times of rest and quiescence. It exactly reverses the effects of the *sympathetic nervous system,* whose function is to activate your body for fight or flight in response to any perceived threat. The sympathetic nervous system increases your heart rate, respiration, blood pressure, and metabolism; tells your muscles to contract; and signals the release of *adrenaline,* a hormone that induces a state of arousal and vigilance. It plays a major role in precipitating stress as well as anxiety. The parasympathetic nervous system signals all of the organs in your body to slow down and tells your muscles to stop contracting. Its function is to return your body to rest after a period of exertion or stress.

People who are anxious or under stress tend to experience high levels of sympathetic nervous system activation much of the time. To use popular expressions, they are "worked up" or "uptight." Even during the times when they begin to calm down, any minor circumstance can set them off once again. After you have been in a state of hyperarousal for a long period of time, the sympathetic nervous system "learns" to be triggered at the slightest provocation. At this point, panic attacks may develop.

At the most basic physiological level, cultivating relaxation means strengthening your predisposition to parasympathetic nervous system activation and decreasing your tendency toward hair-trigger sympathetic nervous system activation. A preference for parasympathetic nervous system arousal is sometimes called *parasympathetic dominance.* The good news is that parasympathetic dominance can be learned, and the exercises in this chapter will help you develop it.

Making Relaxation a Priority

Reordering your priorities is not an easy task. It requires examining values, beliefs, and attitudes that may be so deeply ingrained that you're scarcely aware of them. Given our cultural context, making relaxation a priority that is on par with household chores, career goals, and personal responsibilities may seem particularly unpalatable. After all, the messages we receive from childhood on stress the value of accomplishing, performing, getting it done. It's unlikely that anyone ever encouraged you to learn how to unwind and spend time just being. In addition, modern technological advances have accelerated the pace of life to a dizzying speed. Relaxation, then, requires a deliberate act of will that runs counter to the values and rhythm of our advanced, technological world. No wonder few of us give it a high priority in our daily life.

Challenging as it may be to make relaxation a higher priority, it's well worth the effort if you're trying to live a calmer life that is not dogged by frequent anxiety. It will be easier if you keep in mind that relaxation is not the same as distraction or leisure activities. It is slowing down to a full stop and allowing yourself to enter into a state of deep serenity that you cannot get from going to a movie or playing a computer game.

How much of a priority you make relaxation is ultimately determined by how high a value you place on inner peace. Making time to just be and to cultivate serenity can become the foundation of your life if you so desire. But it requires that you give relaxation a place alongside household responsibilities, work, entertainment, and the pursuit of your other personal goals. Who you believe you are and who you want to be is reflected in where you put your time and energy. When you decide in your innermost self that personal peace is truly important, you'll spend the necessary time to cultivate it.

ATTITUDES THAT UNDERMINE RELAXATION

Below are some common attitudes that undermine relaxation and counterpoints to them.

I have too much to do. There's no time. This is simply another way of saying that relaxation is a low priority. You allocate your time according to your priorities. If relaxation has importance in your life, you'll find the time for it.

Relaxation is too boring. If you feel relaxation is boring, you may have limited acquaintance with how refreshing and revitalizing a truly relaxed state feels. You may not have learned yet to relax deeply. Keep practicing relaxation techniques until you can experience the true benefit of deep relaxation.

I watch TV or read the newspaper. Isn't that relaxation? Relaxation is not the same as distraction. It is an intrinsically pleasurable state that comes from quieting mind and body.

I have to take care of others. Taking time out from caretaking to relax is again a question of priorities. Although it may be challenging at first to make the time, those you care for will benefit when you care for yourself.

I just don't have the discipline. If you feel you don't have the discipline to practice regular periods of relaxation, apply the three-week rule. If you can get yourself to practice deep relaxation every day for three weeks, it will likely become a habit, just like brushing your teeth.

I'm just too tense to unwind. Being too tense to relax may be a problem. One solution is to exercise first, especially to the point of exhaustion. After you discharge excess adrenaline and energy, it may be easier to relax. Another alternative is to have someone give you a good back rub, which is likely to help no matter how tense you feel.

It won't help anyway. If you believe relaxation won't help, you might ask yourself whether you have truly given relaxation a fair chance. If your belief that it won't help is based on previous attempts to relax, perhaps you did not stay with it long enough.

I'm afraid to relax; I might lose control. If this applies to you, start off gently in practicing the relaxation techniques described in this chapter. Try abdominal breathing or progressive muscle relaxation for only two or three minutes at first, and gradually work up to longer time periods. Should you start to feel anxious at any time, simply open your eyes and stop whatever procedure you're practicing until you feel better. Time and practice are the keys to increasing your tolerance for deeper states of relaxation. If your tolerance doesn't improve, it would be helpful to consult a therapist skilled in treating anxiety disorders to assist you in desensitizing yourself to the anxiety you feel about relaxation.

Deep Relaxation

Herbert Benson first described the body's ability to enter into deep relaxation in his 1975 book *The Relaxation Response*. He enumerated a distinct set of physiological changes associated with deep relaxation:

- decrease in heart rate

- decrease in respiration rate

- decrease in blood pressure

- decrease in skeletal muscle tension

- decrease in metabolic rate and oxygen consumption

- decrease in analytical thinking

- increase in skin resistance (the ability of the skin to conduct a mild electrical current)

- increase in alpha wave activity in the brain (of the several types of electrical activity in the brain, alpha waves are consistently associated with subjective states of relaxation)

In short, deep relaxation is a bodily response you can learn. You can train yourself to enter a state of deep relaxation by regularly practicing the relaxation exercises in this chapter.

MAKING DEEP RELAXATION A DAILY PRACTICE MAKES DEEP RELAXATION A DAILY OCCURRENCE

By practicing the relaxation exercises in this chapter daily, you'll begin to achieve a *generalization effect,* which means that a greater sense of relaxation will infuse your daily life. This holds up independent of the quantity and quality of your sleep.

Giving yourself time to relax deeply each day will make it easier to let go and relax at other times, as well as prevent the stresses of daily life from becoming cumulative. In fact, people who relax deeply on a daily basis experience a number of long-term benefits in addition to this generalized relaxation. Such benefits include a reduction of generalized anxiety, an increase in energy level, improved concentration and memory, reduced insomnia, relief from a variety of psychosomatic ailments (such as high blood pressure, ulcers, migraines, and asthma), and increased self-confidence.

Guidelines for Getting the Most out of Relaxation Exercises

The following guidelines will help you to make the most of the relaxation exercises in this chapter. You may want to photocopy these guidelines and keep them handy when you're first learning a relaxation technique.

Practice at least twenty minutes per day. (The exception to this is abdominal breathing, which you should do for five to ten minutes at a time, preferably three times per day.) Two twenty-minute periods are preferable. Once a day is mandatory if you want to make a difference in the quality of your life. You may want to begin your practice with one or two thirty-minute periods. As you gain skill in relaxation techniques, you will find that the amount of time you need to experience deep relaxation will decrease.

Practice in a quiet location where you won't be distracted. Don't permit the phone to ring while you're practicing. Use a fan or air conditioner to block out background noise if necessary.

Practice at regular times. On awakening, before retiring, or before meals are generally the best times. A consistent daily routine will increase the likelihood of generalization effects.

Practice on an empty stomach. Food digestion after meals will tend to disrupt deep relaxation, so practice at least one hour before or one hour after a meal.

Assume a comfortable position. Your entire body, including your head, should be supported. Lying down on a sofa or bed or sitting in a reclining chair are two ways of supporting your body most completely. (When lying down, you may want to place a pillow beneath your knees for further support.) Sitting up is preferable to lying down if you are feeling tired or sleepy. It's advantageous to experience the full depth of the relaxation consciously without going to sleep.

Let your body be unencumbered. Loosen any tight garments and take off shoes, watch, glasses, contact lenses, jewelry, and so on.

Make a decision not to worry about anything. Give yourself permission to put aside the concerns of the day. Allow taking care of yourself and having peace of mind to take precedence over any of your worries. (Remember that success with relaxation depends on giving peace of mind high priority in your overall scheme of values.)

Assume a passive, detached attitude. This is probably the most important element. You want to adopt a let-it-happen attitude and be free of any worry about how well you are performing the technique. Do not try to relax. Do not try to control your body. Do not judge your performance. The point is to let go.

Progressive Muscle Relaxation

Edmund Jacobson (1974), the physician who developed *progressive muscle relaxation* (PMR) in the 1930s, noted that it is impossible for the mind to be anxious when the body is truly relaxed. Although he initially prescribed PMR for reducing blood pressure, it has become a staple technique for treating anxiety. Jacobson discovered that a muscle could be relaxed by first tensing it for a few seconds and then releasing it. Tensing and relaxing a number of different muscle groups throughout the body in succession produces a state of deep relaxation.

PMR involves tensing and relaxing sixteen different muscle groups. The idea is to tense (not strain) each muscle group hard for about ten seconds and then to let go of it suddenly. You then give yourself fifteen to twenty seconds to relax, noticing how the muscle group feels when relaxed in contrast to how it felt when tensed, before going on to the next group of muscles.

If your anxiety is marked by muscle tension and racing thoughts, PMR will probably be especially valuable to you. Tension headaches, backaches, tightness in the jaw or around the eyes, insomnia, high blood pressure, and tension in the back and shoulders all respond to PMR.

GUIDELINES FOR PRACTICING PROGRESSIVE MUSCLE RELAXATION

If you have suffered a muscle injury, consult your doctor before beginning PMR.

When you tense a particular muscle group, do so vigorously, without straining, for seven to ten seconds. You may want to count *one thousand one, one thousand two,* and so on as a way of marking off seconds. Concentrate on what is happening. Feel the buildup of tension in each muscle group. It's often helpful to visualize the particular muscle group being tensed.

When you release the muscles, do so abruptly, and then relax, enjoying the sudden feeling of limpness. Relax for at least fifteen to twenty seconds before going on to the next group of muscles. You might also say to yourself *I am relaxing, Letting go, Let the tension flow away,* or any other relaxing phrase during each relaxation period between successive muscle groups. Allow all the other muscles in your body to remain relaxed, as far as possible, while tensing a particular muscle group. Tense and relax each muscle group once. If a particular area feels especially tight, you can tense and relax it two or three times, waiting about twenty seconds between each cycle.

You might want to record the following exercise on an audiocassette to expedite your early practice sessions. Or you may wish to obtain a professionally made tape of progressive muscle relaxation. Some people always prefer to use a tape, while others have the exercises so well learned after a few weeks of practice that they prefer doing them from memory.

Exercise: Progressive Muscle Relaxation

1. To begin, take three deep breaths, feeling your belly expand with each breath. Inhale and exhale

slowly through your nose each time. As you exhale, imagine that the tension throughout your body begins to flow away.

2. Clench your fists. Hold for seven to ten seconds and then release for fifteen to twenty seconds. Use these same time intervals for all other muscle groups.

3. Tighten your biceps by drawing your forearms up toward your shoulders and "making a muscle" with both arms. Hold . . . and then relax.

4. Tighten your triceps (the muscles on the undersides of your upper arms) by extending your arms out straight and locking your elbows. Hold . . . and then relax.

5. Tense the muscles in your forehead by raising your eyebrows as far as you can. Hold . . . and then relax. Imagine your forehead muscles becoming smooth and limp as they relax.

6. Tense the muscles around your eyes by clenching your eyelids tightly shut. Hold . . . and then relax. Imagine sensations of deep relaxation spreading all around the area of your eyes.

7. Tighten your jaws by opening your mouth widely so that you stretch the muscles around the hinges of your jaw. Hold . . . and then relax. Allow your jaw to hang loose.

8. Tighten the muscles in the back of your neck by pulling your head way back, as if you were going to touch your head to your back (be gentle with this muscle group to avoid injury). Focus only on tensing the muscles in your neck. Hold . . . and then relax. Since this area is often especially tight, it's good to do the tense-relax cycle twice.

9. Take a few deep breaths and tune in to the weight of your head sinking into whatever surface it's resting on.

10. Tighten your shoulders by raising them up as if you were going to touch your ears. Hold . . . and then relax.

11. Tighten the muscles around your shoulder blades by pushing back your shoulders as if you were going to touch them together. Hold the tension in your shoulder blades . . . and then relax. Since this area is often especially tense, you might repeat the tense-relax sequence twice.

12. Tighten the muscles of your chest by taking in a deep breath. Hold for up to ten seconds . . . and then release slowly. Imagine any excess tension in your chest flowing away with the exhalation.

13. Tighten your stomach muscles by sucking your stomach in. Hold . . . and then release. Imagine a wave of relaxation spreading through your abdomen.

14. Tighten your lower back muscles by arching your back. (You can omit this part if you have lower back pain.) Hold . . . and then relax.

15. Tighten your buttock muscles by pulling them together. Hold . . . and then relax. Imagine the muscles in your hips going loose and limp.

16. Squeeze the muscles in your thighs all the way down to your knees. You will probably have to tighten your buttocks along with your thighs, since the thigh muscles attach at the pelvis. Hold . . . and then relax. Feel your thigh muscles smoothing out and relaxing completely.

17. Tighten your calf muscles by pulling your toes toward you (flex carefully to avoid cramps). Hold . . . and then relax.

18. Tighten your feet by curling your toes downward. Hold . . . and then relax.

19. Mentally scan your body for any residual tension. If a particular area remains tense, repeat one or two tense-relax cycles for that group of muscles.

Now imagine a wave of relaxation gradually spreading throughout your body, starting at your head and slowly penetrating every muscle group all the way down to your toes.

Passive Muscle Relaxation

As an alternative to progressive muscle relaxation, you may want to try *passive muscle relaxation,* which does not require actively tensing and relaxing your muscles. Progressive muscle relaxation is a slightly more potent medicine for body tension, but passive muscle relaxation works quite well too.

Exercise: Passive Muscle Relaxation

Use the following script when you practice passive muscle relaxation. You can have someone slowly read it to you, or record it on an audiocassette in your own voice.

Start out by taking two or three deep breaths . . . and let yourself settle back into the chair, the bed, or wherever you happen to be right now . . . making yourself fully comfortable. Let this be a time just for you, putting aside all worries and concerns of the day . . . and making this a time just for you . . . letting each part of your body begin to relax . . . starting with your feet. Just imagine your feet letting go and relaxing right now . . . letting go of any excess tension in your feet. Just imagine it draining away . . . and as your feet are relaxing, imagine relaxation moving up into your calves. Let the muscles in your calves unwind and loosen up and let go . . . allow any tension you're feeling in your calves to just drain away easily and quickly . . . and as your calves are relaxing, allow relaxation to move up into your thighs . . . let the muscles in your thighs unwind and smooth out and relax completely. You might begin to feel your legs from your waist down to your feet becoming more and more relaxed. You might notice your legs becoming heavy as they relax more and more. Continuing now to let the relaxation move into your hips . . . feeling any excess tension in your hips dissolve and flow away. And soon you might allow relaxation to move into your stomach area . . . just letting go of any strain or discomfort in your stomach . . . let it all go right now, imagining deep sensations of relaxation spreading all around your stomach . . . and continuing to allow the relaxation to move up into your chest. All the muscles in your chest can unwind and loosen up and let go. Each time you exhale, you might imagine breathing away any remaining tension in your chest until your chest feels completely relaxed . . . and you find it easy to enjoy the good feeling of relaxation as it deepens and develops throughout your chest, stomach area, and your legs. And shortly, you might allow relaxation to move into your shoulders . . . just letting deep sensations of calmness and relaxation spread all through the muscles of your shoulders . . . allowing your shoulders to drop . . . allowing them to feel completely relaxed. And you might now allow the relaxation in your shoulders to move down into your arms, spreading into your upper arms, down into your elbows and forearms, and finally all the way down to your wrists and hands . . . letting your arms relax . . . enjoying the good feeling of relaxation in your arms

. . . putting aside any worries, any uncomfortable, unpleasant thoughts right now . . . letting yourself be totally in the present moment as you let yourself relax more and more. You can feel relaxation moving into your neck now. All the muscles in your neck just unwind, smooth out, and relax completely. Imagine the muscles in your neck loosening up just like a knotted cord being unraveled. And soon, the relaxation can move into your chin and jaws . . . allowing your jaws to relax . . . letting your jaws loosen up, and as they are relaxing, you can imagine relaxation moving into the area around your eyes. Any tension around your eyes can just dissipate and flow away as you allow your eyes to relax completely. Any eyestrain just dissolves now and your eyes can fully relax. And you let your forehead relax too . . . letting the muscles in your forehead smooth out and relax completely . . . noticing the weight of your head against whatever it's resting on as you allow your entire head to relax completely. Just enjoying the good feeling of relaxation all over . . . letting yourself drift deeper and deeper into quietness and peace . . . getting more and more in touch with that place deep inside of perfect stillness and serenity.

Abdominal Breathing versus Chest Breathing

Shallow, chest-level breathing is a common symptom of anxiety and also an aggravating factor in it. When you breathe from your chest, you have a tendency to slip into one of two anxiety-producing breathing patterns: *underbreathing* or *overbreathing*. If you are underbreathing and not getting enough oxygen to your brain, you may develop a closed-in feeling that becomes progressively more uncomfortable. The sensation of being trapped that prompts many phobic people to want to flee situations—like riding in elevators, waiting in line, or driving in traffic—may in part be due to oxygen starvation from underbreathing (along with the restriction of the ability to move). Overbreathing occurs when you breathe so rapidly that you exhale too much carbon dioxide. This happens especially if you are breathing through your mouth. Often referred to as *hyperventilation,* overbreathing leads to a cluster of uncomfortable symptoms including jitteriness, tingling in your extremities or face, dizziness, disorientation, and even a sense of unreality. If you interpret hyperventilation symptoms as threatening or dangerous (which they aren't), you may well trigger a panic attack.

By contrast, abdominal breathing fosters a sense of calm. It activates your parasympathetic nervous system, which in turn sends an all-is-well message to the rest of your body. Abdominal breathing is the most rapid and direct technique you can use to offset anxiety and relax. Regular daily practice of abdominal breathing will retrain you to breathe more from your diaphragm and less from your chest. The result is that you will feel more relaxed in general. Abdominal breathing can also be used to diffuse anxiety the moment it arises.

The way you know you are doing abdominal breathing is simple: If you place your hand on your stomach, your hand should rise as you inhale and fall as you exhale. Your chest, however, should move very little or not at all. It's best to sit or lie down while practicing abdominal breathing.

GUIDELINES FOR PRACTICING ABDOMINAL BREATHING

By practicing the following two exercises, you'll begin to get into the habit of breathing from your abdomen instead of your chest. Try both the abdominal breathing exercise and the calming breath exercise, but work on mastering abdominal breathing first. When you become proficient in both techniques, choose the one you prefer to practice on a regular basis.

Practice for at least five to ten minutes at a time, three times per day, for at least three weeks. If possible, find regular times each day to do this so that your breathing exercise becomes a habit. With practice you can learn to use these breathing exercises to slow down the physiological reactions that happen when anxiety arises.

Exercise: Abdominal Breathing

1. While sitting or lying down, preferably with your head supported, place one hand on your abdomen, right beneath your rib cage.

2. Inhale slowly and deeply through your nose into the bottom of your lungs (the deepest point in your lungs that you can reach). Your chest should move only slightly, while your stomach rises, pushing your hand up.

3. When you've inhaled fully, pause for a moment and then exhale fully through your nose or your mouth. Be sure to exhale completely. As you exhale, allow yourself to let go, and imagine your entire body going loose and limp. In order to fully relax, take and release ten abdominal breaths. (When you've completed ten breaths, keep practicing abdominal breathing for five to ten minutes more.) Try to keep your breathing smooth and regular throughout, without gulping in air or exhaling suddenly. It will help to slow down your breathing if you slowly count to four on the inhale and then slowly count to four again on the exhale. Use the one-to-four count for at least the first day or two of practicing abdominal breathing. After you've become proficient in slowing down your breathing, you can drop the one-to-four count if you wish. Optional: At this point, you may want to try counting backward from twenty down to one, one count after each exhale.

That is, after the first exhale count *twenty,* after the next *nineteen,* and so on, down to one. Then start over again at twenty and repeat the cycle. Remember to keep your breath slow and regular throughout, inhaling through your nose and exhaling through your nose or mouth. (You may prefer to do simple abdominal breathing without counting down.)

4. Continue to practice abdominal breathing for at least five to ten minutes. If you start to feel light-headed at any time, stop for thirty seconds and then start up again.

Exercise: Calming Breath

1. Breathing from your abdomen, inhale through your nose slowly to a count of five.

2. Pause and hold your breath to a slow count of five.

3. Exhale slowly, through your nose or mouth, to a slow count of five (or six, seven, or eight, if it takes you longer). Be sure to exhale fully.

4. When you've exhaled completely, take two breaths in your normal rhythm, then repeat the first three steps in the cycle above.

5. Keep up the exercise for five minutes. This should involve going through at least ten cycles of *in* five, *hold* five, *out* five. As you continue the exercise, you may notice that you can count higher than five, or count higher when you exhale than when you inhale. If these variations in your counting do occur, simply allow them to, continuing with the exercise for five minutes. Remember to take two normal breaths between each cycle. If you start to feel light-headed while practicing this exercise, stop for thirty

seconds, breathe normally, and then start again. Throughout the exercise, keep your breathing smooth and regular, without gulping in breaths or breathing out suddenly.

6. Optional: Each time you exhale, you may wish to say *Relax, Calm, Let go,* or any other relaxing word or phrase silently to yourself. Allow your whole body to let go as you do this. If you keep this up each time you practice, eventually just saying your relaxing word by itself will bring on a mild state of relaxation.

Guided Visualization

Guided visualization is a method of deliberately using mental imagery to modify your behavior, the way you feel, and even your internal physiological state. You can consciously create visualizations as a preventative measure against anxiety. When you practice guided visualization, you will close your eyes and imagine yourself in a calming scene. Taking on this new role in a mental movie designed to induce serenity rather than suspense can go a long way to reduce your anxiety symptoms. Below are two guided visualizations you can use to relax your mind when you feel tense or worried.

Visualization itself is inherently relaxing, but you may find it helpful to relax your body using abdominal breathing for a minute or two before you begin to practice visualization. When you are relaxed, you're able to experience the images more vividly, and thus they are likely to have a more profound effect. So that you have the optimal chance to relax, it is useful to record guided visualizations on tape, either in your own voice or by asking someone else to make the recording (naturally, you should choose someone whose voice sounds pleasant to you). After you've gone through the visualization a number of times on tape, you may recall it so well that you can do it on your own, or you may prefer to continue using the tape indefinitely.

GUIDELINES FOR PRACTICING GUIDED VISUALIZATION

• Get into a comfortable position, free of encumbrances and with your head supported. Be sure that your environment is quiet and free from distractions. Give yourself time to relax before undertaking a guided visualization. To this end, you can use progressive muscle relaxation or abdominal breathing for a few minutes before you start.

• At the conclusion of your relaxing visualization, bring yourself back to an alert state of mind with the following statement, which you can record at the end of your visualization tape:

Now, in a moment you can begin to come back to an alert, wakeful state of mind. Pay attention as I count from one up to five. When I get up to five, you can open your eyes and feel awake, alert, and refreshed. One . . . gradually beginning to come back to an alert, wakeful state. Two . . . more and more awake. Three . . . beginning to move your hands and feet as you become more alert. Four . . . almost back to a fully alert state. And five . . . opening your eyes now, finding yourself fully awake, alert, and refreshed.

• After finishing with your visualization, get up and walk around a bit until you feel fully alert and grounded. Allow at least ten minutes to pass before driving a car or engaging in any other activity that requires complex coordination.

Exercise: A Guided Visualization of the Beach

You're walking down a long wooden stairway to a beautiful, expansive beach. It looks almost deserted and stretches off into the distance as far as you can see. The sand is very fine and light . . . almost white in appearance. You step onto the sand in your bare feet and rub it between your toes. It feels so good to walk slowly along this beautiful beach. The roaring sound of the surf is so soothing that you can just let go of anything on your mind. You're watching the waves ebb and flow . . . they are slowly coming in . . . breaking over each other . . . and then slowly flowing back out again. The ocean itself is a very beautiful shade of blue . . . a shade of blue that is so relaxing just to look at. You look out over the surface of the ocean all the way to the horizon and then follow the horizon as far as you can see, noticing how it bends slightly downward as it follows the curvature of the earth. As you scan the ocean you can see, many miles offshore, a tiny sailboat skimming along the surface of the water. And all these sights help you to just let go and relax even more. As you continue walking down the beach, you become aware of the fresh, salty smell of the sea air. You take in a deep breath . . . breathe out . . . and feel very refreshed and even more relaxed. Overhead you notice two seagulls flying out to sea . . . looking very graceful as they soar into the wind . . . and you imagine how you might feel yourself if you had the freedom to fly. You find yourself settling into a deep state of relaxation as you continue walking down the beach. You feel the sea breeze blowing gently against your cheek and the warmth of the sun overhead penetrating your neck and shoulders. The warm, liquid sensation of the sun just relaxes you even more . . . and you're beginning to feel perfectly content on this beautiful beach. It's such a lovely day. In a moment, up ahead, you see a comfortable-looking beach chair. Slowly, you begin to approach the beach chair . . . and when you finally reach it, you sit back and settle in. Lying back in this comfortable beach chair, you let go and relax even more, drifting even deeper into relaxation. In a little while you might close your eyes and just listen to the sound of the surf, the unending cycle of waves ebbing and flowing. And the rhythmic sound of the surf carries you even deeper . . . deeper still . . . into a wonderful state of quietness and peace.

Exercise: A Guided Visualization of the Forest

You're walking along a path deep in the forest. All around you there are tall trees . . . pine, fir, redwood, oak . . . try to see them. The rushing sound of the wind blowing through the treetops is so soothing, allowing you to let go. You can smell the rich dampness of the forest floor, the smell of earth, and new seedlings, and rotting leaves. Now you look up through the treetops until you can see a light blue sky. You notice how high the sun is in the sky. As the sun enters the canopy of the treetops, it splinters into rays that penetrate through the trees to the forest floor. You're watching the intricate patterns of light and dark created as the light filters down through the trees. The forest feels like a great primeval cathedral . . . filling you with a sense of peace and reverence for all living things. Off in the distance, you can hear the sound of rushing water echoing through the forest. It gets louder as you approach, and before long you are at the edge of a mountain stream. You're looking at the stream, noticing how clear and sparkling the water is. Imagine sitting down and making yourself very comfortable. You might sit down on a flat rock up against a tree, or you might even decide to lie down on a grassy slope. You can see the mountain stream creating rapids as it moves, rushing around a variety of large and small rocks.

These rocks are many shades of brown, gray, and white, and some are covered with moss. You can see the sparkling water rushing over some and around others, making whirlpools and eddies. The rushing sound of the water is so peaceful that you can just let yourself drift . . . relaxing more and more. You take in a deep breath of fresh air and breathe out, finding the subtle smells of the forest very refreshing. As you let yourself sink into the soft bed of grass or dead leaves or fragrant pine needles beneath you, you let go of any strains or concerns . . . allowing the sights, sounds, and smells of this beautiful forest to fill you with a deep sense of peace.

Pacing

While PMR, breathing exercises, and visualizations are useful tools for promoting relaxation, they are only part of the overall formula for it. Setting the right pace for your life is equally important. Like many anxiety sufferers, you may set too fast a pace for yourself and allow outside influences, such as societal pressure to achieve, to dictate the rate at which you live. Another common pitfall is looking to others to determine how busy you should be. Using other people's output or activity level as a benchmark for what you should accomplish is akin to buying a suit according to someone else's measurements and expecting a tailored fit.

Pacing means living at *your* optimal rate. Routinely cramming in more activity than your body can handle leads to exhaustion, stress, and possibly illness, while doing too little yields boredom and self-absorption. Achieving your optimal pace requires listening to your body's cues to determine how many activities you should take on in a given day. Acknowledging and respecting your body's need for rest and rejuvenation will help you live at the speed best suited to you. In a society that encourages competition and reveres accomplishment, it's easy to become deaf to your body's signals that it needs rest. Paying closer attention to these signals will enhance your overall sense of relaxation.

MINIBREAKS

Taking a five- or ten-minute minibreak every hour or two can be quite helpful if you're trying to slow down. Minibreaks can be especially effective if you take them between activities. For example, after commuting in the morning, take a short break before beginning work. Or after cooking a meal, take a short break before sitting down to eat. During your break, you might practice abdominal breathing, meditate, take a stroll, do a few yoga stretches, or do anything else that helps you to reenergize, relax, and clear your mind. Ironically, you may find that you actually get more done when you interperse short breaks into your daily activities. You will bring more energy and clarity to each thing you do.

DOWNTIME

Taking downtime means deliberately spending a period of time away from work and other responsibilities to relax and enjoy yourself. Without downtime, everyday stresses become cumulative and take a toll on your well-being. Downtime gives you a break from stress and an opportunity to replenish your energy.

Optimally, you should take the following amounts of downtime: one hour per day, one day per week, and one week every twelve to sixteen weeks. If taking four weeks off per year isn't an option, try to take at least a few days every three to four months, even if they are unpaid. During these periods you should disengage from any work-related tasks, put aside those responsibilities that can be postponed, and choose not to answer the phone unless you know it's someone you enjoy hearing from.

REST TIME, RECREATION TIME, AND RELATIONSHIP TIME

There are three kinds of downtime: *rest time, recreation time,* and *relationship time.* Each of these plays an essential role in a more relaxed lifestyle, and it's important to make time for all three. Often recreation and relationship time can be combined, but rest time should be used for just that and nothing else.

Rest time is time when you set aside all activities and just allow yourself to be. You stop action and let yourself fully rest. Rest time might involve lying on the couch and doing nothing, quietly meditating, sitting in your recliner and listening to peaceful music, soaking in a hot tub, or taking a catnap in the middle of the workday. Rest time is fundamentally passive. It's when you allow yourself to stop doing and accomplishing and just be. Since the rest of your time is focused on producing and accomplishing goals, rest time is a necessary counterpoint. When you're under stress, one hour of rest time per day, separate from the time you sleep, is optimal.

Unlike rest time, recreation time is active. It involves engaging in activities that help to "re-create" and replenish your energy. Recreation time brightens and uplifts your spirits. In essence, it's doing anything that you experience as fun or play. Such activities might include puttering in the garden, reading a novel, seeing a special movie, going on a hike, playing volleyball, taking a short trip, baking a loaf of bread, or fishing. You can take time for recreation during the work week, but it's most important on your days off from work. Such time can be spent either alone or with someone else.

Relationship time is time when you put aside your private goals and responsibilities in order to enjoy being with another person, or, in some cases, with several people. The focus of relationship time is to honor your relationship with your partner, children, extended family members, friends, pets, and so on, and forget about your individual pursuits for a while. If you have a family, relationship time needs to be allocated equitably between time alone with your spouse, time alone with your children, and time when the entire family gets together. If you have a partner but no children, time needs to be allocated between your partner and friends. When you slow down and make time to be with others, you're not as likely to neglect your own basic needs for intimacy, touching, affection, validation, and support. Meeting these basic needs is absolutely vital to your well-being. Without sufficient time devoted to important relationships, you will likely suffer, and the people you most care about are bound to as well.

How can you allow for more downtime (of all three kinds) in your life? It requires a genuine commitment to leading a more relaxed and easy lifestyle, apart from what the neighbors and the rest of the world may be doing. Deliberately making time for rest, recreation, and relationships may be challenging at first, but tends to become easier and more rewarding as time goes on. For some people, it translates into a fundamental decision to make earning money less important and a simpler, more balanced lifestyle more important. Before you think about leaving your present job, however, consider how you can shift your values toward placing more emphasis on the process of life (how you live) as opposed to accomplishments and productivity (what you actually do) within your current life situation. Take some time to reflect on how you might allocate more time for each of the three types of downtime. Write down your ideas for including more downtime in your life.

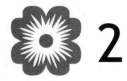 2

Exercise: A Natural Outlet for Anxiety

There are few images that better symbolize daily life in contemporary America than a seated individual. Most of us sit at work, sit during our leisure activities, and sit when we travel. The technological advances and material abundance that began in the twentieth century have translated into a lifestyle of unprecedented inactivity. The problem is that our physical evolution doesn't keep pace with our social evolution. The human body evolved in a physically exacting environment, so even though it may no longer be necessary for survival, we are prewired to be active. Inactivity takes a steep toll on physical and mental well-being. It is a contributing factor in obesity, hypertension, depression, and, yes, anxiety.

A Natural Outlet for Anxiety

When anxiety hits, your body goes into fight-or-flight mode. That means that your sympathetic nervous system is activated and a surge of adrenaline is released. The message your body gets is *Get ready to move fast!* Remaining inactive in the face of this state of activation usually intensifies your symptoms.

Exercise is a natural outlet for anxiety. When you become physically active the minute your anxiety symptoms begin, you satisfy your body's need to act and tell your mind that the danger has passed and it can turn off the alarm signals. If anxiety takes hold in a place where you cannot move easily, like in a grocery store line or while driving in traffic, make a promise to yourself to get active as soon as possible.

The Preventative Value of Exercise

Like many of the techniques discussed in this book, exercise prevents as well as contains anxiety. One reason for this is that exercise has a clearly established ability to raise the level of *serotonin* in the brain and to increase the activity of serotonin in the cerebral cortex. Serotonin is a neurotransmitter, one of the chemicals in your brain that facilitates transmission of nerve signals. Increased serotonin is associated with amelioration of all of the anxiety disorders, which is why many people tend to improve after taking *selective serotonin reuptake inhibitor* (SSRI) medications.

Exercise also counters several of the physiological factors that underlie anxiety, which is why people who exercise regularly tend to have less frequent and milder episodes of anxiety. Exercise brings about:

- reduced skeletal muscle tension, which is largely responsible for your feelings of being tense or "uptight"

- more rapid metabolism of excess *adrenaline* and *thyroxin* in the bloodstream (the presence of these hormones tends to keep you in a state of arousal and vigilance)

- a discharge of pent-up frustration, which can aggravate phobic or panic reactions

Exercise results in several psychological benefits that may also help reduce anxiety:

- increased subjective feelings of well-being

- reduced dependence on alcohol and drugs

- reduced insomnia

- improved concentration and memory

- reduced depression

- increased self-esteem

- greater sense of control over stress and anxiety

Additional physiological benefits of exercise include:

- enhanced oxygenation of the blood and brain, which increases alertness and concentration

- stimulation of the production of *endorphins,* natural substances in your brain that resemble morphine both chemically and in their effects, increasing your sense of well-being

- improved circulation

- improved digestion and utilization of food

- improved elimination (from skin, lungs, and bowels)

- decreased cholesterol levels

- decreased blood pressure

- weight loss, as well as appetite suppression in many cases

- improved blood sugar regulation (in the case of hypoglycemia)

Are You Ready for an Exercise Program?

There are certain physical conditions that may limit the amount and intensity of exercise you should undertake. Ask yourself the eight questions below before launching a program of regular exercise. If your answer to any of them is yes, be sure to consult your physician before beginning an exercise routine. He or she may recommend a program of restricted or supervised exercise appropriate to your needs.

1. Has your physician ever said you have heart trouble?

2. Do you frequently have pains in your heart or chest?

3. Do you often feel faint or have spells of dizziness?

4. Has your physician ever told you that you have a bone or joint problem (such as arthritis) that has been or might be aggravated by exercise?

5. Has a physician ever said that your blood pressure was too high?

6. Do you have diabetes?

7. Are you over forty years old and unaccustomed to vigorous exercise?

8. Is there a physical reason not mentioned here why you should not undertake an exercise program?

If you answered no to all of the above questions, you can be reasonably assured that you are ready to start an exercise program. Begin slowly and increase your activity gradually over a period of weeks. If you are over forty and unaccustomed to exercise, plan to see your doctor for a physical exam before undertaking an exercise program. It might also be helpful to have a support person exercise with you initially. If you feel phobic about exercise, a program of gradual exposure, starting with just a few minutes and working up gradually to longer time periods, will help you get used to it.

Optimizing the Anxiety-Reducing Effects of Exercise

Exercise needs to be of sufficient regularity, intensity, and duration to have a significant impact on anxiety. The following guidelines will help you get the most benefit from your exercise program:

- Ideally, you should engage in an aerobic exercise. Common forms of aerobic exercise include fast walking (for an hour), jogging, vigorous cycling, freestyle swimming, aerobic dancing, and jumping rope.

- Exercise four to five times per week for twenty to thirty minutes.

- Optimal intensity for aerobic exercise is a heart rate of *(220 – your age) x 0.75* for at least ten minutes.

Aerobic Pulse Ranges by Age

Age	Pulse (Heart) Rate
20–29	145–164
30–39	138–156
40–49	130–148
50–59	122–140
60–69	116–132

- Avoid exercising only once per week. Engaging in infrequent spurts of exercise is stressful to your body and generally does more harm than good. (Walking is an exception.)

Exercise for Your Needs

Which forms of exercise you select depends upon your objectives. For reducing anxiety, aerobic exercise is typically the most effective. Aerobic exercise requires sustained activity of your larger muscles. It reduces skeletal muscle tension and increases cardiovascular conditioning, the capacity of your circulatory system to deliver oxygen to your tissues and cells with greater efficiency. Regular aerobic exercise will reduce stress and increase your stamina.

Beyond aerobic fitness, you may have other objectives in taking up exercise. If increased muscle strength is important, you may want to include weight lifting or isometric exercise in your program. (If you have a heart condition or angina, you should probably not engage in weight lifting or bodybuilding.) Exercise that involves stretching, such as dancing or yoga, is ideal for developing muscular flexibility and is a good complement to aerobic exercise. If you want to lose weight, jogging or cycling is probably most effective. If discharging aggression and frustration is important, you might try competitive sports. Finally, if you just want to get out into nature, then hiking or gardening would be appropriate. Vigorous hiking (as done by the Sierra Club, for example) can increase both strength and endurance.

Many people find it helpful to vary the type of exercise they do. Doing two or more different forms of exercise on alternate days is sometimes referred to as *cross-training*. This gives you the opportunity to develop a more balanced state of fitness by exercising different muscle groups. Popular combinations involve doing an aerobic type of exercise (such as jogging or cycling) three to four times a week and a socializing exercise (such as golf), or a bodybuilding exercise, twice a week. Maintaining a program with two distinct types of exercise prevents either from becoming too boring.

Following are brief descriptions of some of the more common types of aerobic exercise. Each type has its advantages and possible drawbacks.

RUNNING

For many years, jogging or running has been the most popular form of aerobic exercise, perhaps because of its convenience. The only equipment you need is running shoes, and in many cases you need only step out your door to begin. Running is one of the best forms of exercise for losing weight, as it burns calories quickly. Numerous studies have shown its benefits for depression, as it raises both endorphin and serotonin levels in the brain. Running decreases anxiety by metabolizing excess adrenaline and releasing skeletal muscle tension. A three-mile jog (approximately thirty minutes) four or five times per week can go a long way toward diminishing your vulnerability to anxiety. Work up to a pace of one mile every twelve minutes.

The downside to running is that over a period of time, it can increase your risk of injury. In particular, if you run on hard surfaces, the constant shock to your joints can lead to foot, knee, or back problems. You can minimize your risk of injury by:

- Getting proper shoes—those that minimize shock to your joints.

- Running on soft surfaces—preferably grass, dirt, a track, or a hardened beach. Avoid concrete if possible; asphalt is okay if you have good shoes and don't run every day.

- Warming up before you begin. Try doing a minute or two of very slow jogging.

- Alternating jogging with other forms of exercise. Avoid jogging every day.

If running outdoors is a problem because of weather, lack of a soft surface, smog, or traffic, you may want to invest in an automatic treadmill. To make this less boring, put it in front of your TV or VCR.

SWIMMING

Swimming is an especially good exercise because it uses so many different muscles throughout the body. Doctors usually recommend swimming to people with musculoskeletal problems, injuries, or arthritis, because it minimizes shock to the joints. It does not promote weight loss to the same degree as running, but it will help firm up your body.

For aerobic-level conditioning, it's best to swim freestyle for twenty to thirty minutes, preferably four or five times per week. For moderate, relaxing exercise, breaststroke is an enjoyable alternative. As a rule, it's best to work out in a heated pool where the water temperature is seventy-five to eighty degrees.

The major downside with swimming is that many pools are heavily chlorinated. This may be quite irritating to your eyes, skin, or hair, as well as the membranes in your upper respiratory passages. You can counter some of this by wearing goggles and a nose plug. If you're fortunate, you may be able to find a pool that uses hydrogen peroxide or bubbled-in ozone as a disinfectant. If the pool you use is chlorinated, it's a good idea to soap off in a shower afterward.

CYCLING

Cycling has become a very popular form of aerobic exercise in recent years. While having many of the same benefits as jogging, it's less damaging to your joints. To achieve aerobic conditioning, cycling needs to be done vigorously—approximately fifteen miles per hour or more on a flat surface. When the weather is good, cycling can be quite enjoyable, especially if you have beautiful surroundings with little traffic or a designated bike trail. If weather precludes cycling, you can use a stationary bike indoors, possibly in front of your TV or VCR.

If you want to take up outdoor cycling, you'll need to make an initial investment in a good bike. You may want to borrow someone else's bike until you feel ready to spend several hundred dollars. Make sure the bike you purchase is designed and sized correctly for your body, or it may cause you problems. A well-cushioned seat is a good investment.

When you undertake cycling, give yourself a few months to work up to a fifteen-mile-per-hour cruising speed, that is, a mile every four minutes. One hour of cycling three to five times per week is sufficient. Be sure to wear a helmet, and try to avoid riding at night.

AEROBICS CLASSES

Most aerobics classes consist of warm-up stretches and aerobic exercises led by an instructor. These are usually done to music. Classes are generally offered by health clubs, with various levels for beginning, intermediate, and advanced participants. They come under many names, though a couple of recent favorites are *body pump* and *spinning*, which work to increase aerobic fitness as well as strength and endurance. Since certain of the exercises can be traumatic to joints, try to find a low-impact aerobics class. The structured format of an aerobics class may be an excellent way to motivate you to exercise. If you are self-motivated and prefer to stay at home, there are many good aerobics videos available.

If you decide to do aerobic exercises, be sure to obtain good shoes that stabilize your feet, absorb shock, and minimize twisting. It's best to do these exercises on a wooden surface and to avoid thick carpets, if possible. About forty-five minutes to an hour of exercise (including warm-up) three to five times per week is sufficient.

WALKING

Walking has advantages over all other forms of exercise. First, it does not require training—you already know how to do it. Second, it requires no equipment other than a pair of shoes and can be done virtually anywhere—even in a shopping mall, if necessary. The chances of injury are less than for any other type of exercise. Finally, it's the most natural form of activity. All of us are naturally inclined to walk. Until society became sedentary, walking was an integral part of life.

Walking for relaxation and distraction is one thing; doing it for aerobic conditioning is another. To make walking aerobic, aim for about one hour at a brisk enough pace to cover three miles. A twenty- or thirty-minute walk is generally not enough to obtain aerobic-level conditioning. If you make walking your regular form of exercise, do it four to five times per week, preferably outdoors. If you feel an hour of brisk walking is not enough of a workout, try adding hand weights or finding an area with hills. Indoor treadmills can be adjusted to make walking aerobic.

To get the most benefit out of walking, focus on good posture. If it feels natural to allow your arms to swing opposite to the stride of your legs, you'll be getting *cross-lateral conditioning,* which helps to integrate the left and right hemispheres of your brain. Good walking shoes are also important. Look for padded insoles, a good arch, and firm support of the heel.

Once you can comfortably walk three or four miles without stopping, consider taking hiking trips—day or overnight—in county, state, or national parks. Hiking outdoors can revitalize your soul as much as it does your body.

Exercise Should Be (Gasp!) Fun

Exercise should be interesting and fun; it's important that you make it interesting early on so that you keep it up. There are several ways to do this. If you're not limited to being indoors, try to get outside, preferably in an attractive natural setting such as a park or, even better, the countryside. If you're doing a solo-type exercise such as swimming, cycling, or jogging, see if you can find a companion to go with you at least sometimes. If you need to exercise indoors because of personal limitations or climate, play music or watch a video while you're on your stationary bike or treadmill. Some people actually learn foreign languages while exercising!

"The Dog Ate My Running Shoes"

If you are able to come up with a seemingly endless string of excuses to get out of exercising, you are not alone. This does not mean, however, that you should allow yourself to succumb to them. Exercise is an essential component of natural anxiety relief, not an adjunct to it. If you combine regular, aerobic exercise with a program of regular, deep relaxation, you are undoubtedly going to experience a substantial reduction in your anxiety, whether panic attacks or everyday worry. Exercise and deep relaxation are the two methods *most effective* for altering a hereditary predisposition to anxiety—that part of your anxiety that was prewired rather than learned. It is helpful to remind yourself of this if you find excuses taking the place of exercise.

EXCUSES, EXCUSES, EXCUSES

Below are some common excuses for not exercising and counterpoints to them.

"I don't have enough time." What you are really saying is that you're not willing to make time. You aren't assigning enough importance to the increased fitness, well-being, and improved control over anxiety you will surely gain from exercise. The problem is not a matter of time but one of priorities.

"I feel too tired to exercise." One solution is to exercise before going to work—or on your lunch break—rather than at the end of the day. If this is simply impossible, don't give up. What many nonexercisers fail to realize is that moderate exercise can actually *overcome* fatigue. Many people exercise in spite of feeling tired and find that they feel rejuvenated and reenergized afterward. Things will get easier once you get past the initial inertia of starting to exercise.

"Exercise is boring—it's no fun." Is it really true that *all* the activities listed earlier are boring to you? Have you tried out all of them? It may be that you need to find someone to exercise with in order to have more fun. Or perhaps you need to go back and forth between two different types of exercise to stimulate your interest. Exercise can begin to feel wonderful after a few months, when it becomes inherently rewarding, even if it seemed difficult initially.

"It's too inconvenient to go out somewhere to exercise." This is really no problem, as there are several ways to get vigorous exercise in the comfort of your home. Stationary bicycles and powered treadmills have become very popular, and twenty minutes per day on one will give you a good workout. If this seems boring, try listening to a portable CD or tape player with headphones or place your stationary bike or treadmill in front of the TV. Aerobic exercise at home is convenient and fun if you have a VCR. Other indoor activities include jumping on a rebounder, calisthenics, using a rowing machine, or using a universal gym with adjustable weights. There are also early-morning exercise programs on TV. If you can't afford exercise equipment or a VCR, just put on some wild music and dance for twenty minutes. In short, it's quite possible to maintain an adequate exercise program without leaving your home.

"Exercise causes a buildup of lactic acid. Doesn't that cause panic attacks?" It is true that exercise increases the production of lactic acid, and lactic acid can promote panic attacks in some people who are already prone to them. However, regular exercise also increases *oxygen turnover* in your body. Oxygen turnover is the capacity of your body to oxidize substances it doesn't need, including lactic acid. Any increase in lactic acid produced by exercise will be offset by your body's increased capacity to remove it. The net effect of regular exercise is an overall *reduction* in your body's tendency to accumulate lactic acid.

"I'm over forty, and that's too old to start exercising." Unless your doctor gives you a clear medical reason for not exercising, age is never a valid excuse. With patience and persistence, it is possible to get into excellent physical shape at almost any age. Consider the many sixty- and seventy-year-olds who participate in triathlons.

"I'm too overweight and out of shape," or **"I'm afraid I'll have a heart attack if I stress my body by exercising vigorously."** *If you have physical reasons to worry about stressing your heart, be sure to design your exercise program with the help of your physician.* Vigorous walking is a safe exercise for virtually everyone and is considered by some physicians to be the ideal exercise, as it rarely causes muscle or bone injuries. Swimming is also a safe bet if you're out of shape or overweight. Be sensible and realistic in the exercise program you choose. The important thing is to be consistent and committed, whether your program involves walking for one hour every day or training for a marathon.

"I've tried exercise before and it didn't work." The question to ask here is why it didn't work. Did you start off too hard and fast? Did you get bored? Did you balk at the initial aches and pains? Did you feel lonely exercising by yourself? Perhaps it is time for you to give yourself another chance to discover all the physical and psychological benefits of a regular exercise program.

 3

Nurture Body and Mind with a Healthy Diet

Although in recent years much has been written about the connection between food and mood, many of us still don't take diet into consideration when we think about anxiety. Yet a healthy, balanced diet is an important element in any plan to overcome anxiety and achieve wellness. That's because there are foods that promote calmness and mood stability, and, by the same token, there are foods that stoke anxiety and stress. Have you thought about the connection between your intake of sugar and your anxiety? Or about the role that caffeine plays in your symptoms? Did you know that eating an insufficient amount of protein can aggravate anxiety? In this chapter you'll learn the basics of eating a diet that promotes tranquillity and overall well-being.

Three Dietary Culprits

When you're ready to shift your diet to one that nurtures calmness, begin by considering how you can minimize the impact of the three dietary factors most responsible for stirring anxiety: excessive caffeine intake, excessive sugar consumption, and eating foods to which you are allergic. It may be a challenge to limit your intake of caffeine and sugar, especially if you're in the habit of consuming too much of these substances, but doing so will give you more control over your anxiety and contribute to better overall health. Identifying and eliminating foods to which you are allergic can be tough because they are often the foods you crave the most, yet this is well worth the effort too.

CAFFEINE

If we were to make a most-wanted list of the worst dietary triggers of anxiety, caffeine would have to be at the top. That's because caffeine has a directly stimulating effect on several systems in your body. It increases the level of the neurotransmitter *norepinephrine* in your brain, which in turn causes you to feel alert and awake. It increases sympathetic nervous system activity and triggers an adrenaline release, just as stress does. Caffeine also depletes vitamin B_1 *(thiamine),* which is one of the so-called antistress vitamins. Caffeine's place on our most-wanted list would be well deserved.

Daily caffeine intake. Anyone prone to anxiety should reduce total caffeine consumption to less than sixty milligrams per day, which equals about a cup of instant coffee or a cup of regular tea. Remember that caffeine is not just found in coffee, but is in many types of tea, soft drinks, chocolate, cocoa, and over-the-counter drugs too. If you were to stay within the sixty-milligram limit, one cup of instant coffee or one diet cola beverage per day would equal your maximum consumption. Stimulants like *ephedrine* and *pseudoephedrine* mimic the effects of caffeine and should also be avoided.

Caffeine Content of Some Commonly Used Products

Hot Beverage	Caffeine per Cup
Coffee, drip	146 mg
Coffee, instant	66 mg
Coffee, percolated	110 mg
Cocoa	13 mg
Decaffeinated coffee	4 mg
Loose tea, five-minute brew	40 mg
Teabag, five-minute brew	46 mg
Teabag, one-minute brew	28 mg

Soft Drink	Caffeine per 12-Ounce Can
Coca-Cola	65 mg
Diet Dr Pepper	54 mg
Dr Pepper	61 mg
Mountain Dew	55 mg
Pepsi-Cola	43 mg
Tab	49 mg

Over-the-Counter Drug	Caffeine per Tablet
Anacin	32 mg
Caffedrine	200 mg
Empirin	32 mg
Excedrin	65 mg
Midol	132 mg
No-Doz	100 mg
Vanquish	33 mg
Vivarin	200 mg

Other	
Chocolate	25 mg per medium-size candy bar

Caffeine sensitivity. Some of us are more sensitive to the effects of caffeine than others. If you are sensitive, it probably doesn't take more than a cup of tea or a single cola to give you the jitters, and perhaps even a small amount of caffeine leaves you sleepless at night or triggers a panic attack. Some people can trace their first panic attack to excessive intake of caffeine. If you are highly sensitive to caffeine's effects, you would probably do well to avoid it altogether. If you're less sensitive, you may have to experiment a little to see what your optimal caffeine intake is, although for most anxiety sufferers this turns out to be no more than fifty milligrams a day.

Caffeine withdrawal. As with any addictive drug, chronic caffeine consumption leads to increased tolerance and a potential for withdrawal symptoms. If you have been drinking five cups of coffee a day and abruptly cut down to one a day, you may have withdrawal reactions including fatigue, depression, and headaches. It's better to taper off gradually over a period of a month or two. Some people like to substitute decaffeinated coffee, which has about four milligrams of caffeine per cup, while others substitute herbal teas.

SUGAR

The average American consumes about 120 *pounds* of sugar a year! If we were living prior to the twentieth century, it would be logical to infer from this that the average American is exceedingly wealthy. That's because prior to the twentieth century, the only people who could afford such an indulgence were the very rich.

Today sugar is a virtual staple of the American diet. In fact, for many of us, a normal day includes one or two desserts. And sugar is found not just in the dessert foods like cookies and cake but in cereal, salad dressings, processed meat, and other foods. Add to that the regular consumption of high-sugar sodas and sugar-sweetened tea and coffee, and you get a rate of sugar consumption that is unprecedented in human history. Not surprisingly, then, our bodies are not adapted to handle the barrage of sugar we regularly face.

Excessive sugar consumption can create a chronic dysfunction in sugar metabolism. For some people, this dysfunction can lead to excessively high levels of blood sugar, or to diabetes, which became dramatically more prevalent in the twenty-first century. For an even larger number of people, the problem is just the opposite: their blood sugar level periodically drops below normal, a condition called *hypoglycemia.*

Hypoglycemia

What comes to mind when you read the following list of symptoms?

- light-headedness

- mental confusion or disorientation

- trembling

- feelings of unsteadiness or weakness

- irritability

- heart palpitations

Did you think *panic attack?* If so, you may be surprised to know that these are also symptoms of hypoglycemia. Hypoglycemia symptoms tend to crop up when blood sugar drops below fifty to sixty milliliters per milliliter, or when it plummets from a high level to a low level. Many people with hypoglycemia find that their "panic" disappears after they have something to eat. If you have any of the above symptoms three or four hours after a meal, and they go away as soon as you have something to eat, you should speak to your doctor about the possibility that you have hypoglycemia. The majority of people with anxiety problems find that their panic or anxiety reactions do not necessarily correlate with bouts of low blood sugar. Still, hypoglycemia often aggravates both generalized anxiety and panic attacks that have other causes.

Hypoglycemia can be formally diagnosed through the *six-hour glucose tolerance test*. After a twelve-hour fast, you drink a highly concentrated sugar solution. Your blood sugar is then measured at half-hour intervals over a six-hour period. You will likely get a positive result on this test if you have a moderate to severe problem with hypoglycemia. Unfortunately, many milder cases of hypoglycemia are missed by the test. It's quite possible to have subjective symptoms of low blood sugar and test negative on a glucose tolerance test. Any of the following subjective symptoms are suggestive of hypoglycemia:

- Feeling anxious, light-headed, weak, or irritable three or four hours after a meal (or in the middle of the night), and feeling relief within a few minutes of eating.

- Getting a "high" feeling from consuming sugar, which changes to a depressed, irritable, or spacey feeling twenty to thirty minutes later.

- Experiencing anxiety, restlessness, or even palpitations and panic in the early morning hours, between 4:00 and 7:00 A.M. (Your blood sugar is lowest in the early morning because you have fasted all night.)

Fortunately, it's quite possible to overcome problems with low blood sugar by making several important dietary changes and taking certain supplements.

Dietary changes for hypoglycemia. The following dietary changes would be helpful if you suffer from hypoglycemia:

- Try to eliminate all types of sugar from your diet. This includes foods that obviously contain white sugar or sucrose, such as candy, ice cream, cake, and soft drinks. It also includes subtler forms of sugar such as honey, brown sugar, corn syrup, corn sweeteners, molasses, maltose, dextrose, and fructose. Be sure to read labels on any and all processed foods to detect these various forms of sugar. If you must have a sweet, have something small right after a meal.

- Substitute fruits (other than dried fruits, which are too concentrated in sugar) for sweets. Avoid fruit juices, or use just a splash to flavor water.

- Reduce simple carbohydrates such as pasta, refined cereals, potato or corn chips, and white bread. Substitute instead *complex carbohydrates,* such as whole-grain breads and cereals, brown rice, and vegetables, which have a low *glycemic index.* The glycemic index indicates the rate at which blood sugar rises after a person eats a particular food. The lower the food on the index, the more gradual the rise in blood sugar, and the less stress it causes the body. (For more information on the glycemic index, see the books by Barry Sears and Andrew Weil in the resources and references in the back of this book.)

- Have a complex carbohydrate and protein snack (such as whole-grain crackers and cheese, whole-grain toast with tuna, or nuts such as almonds or cashews) halfway between meals—around 10:30 or 11:00 A.M. and especially around 4:00 or 5:00 P.M. Avoid sweets between meals. If you awaken early in the morning, you may also find that a small snack will help you to get back to sleep for a couple of hours. As an alternative to snacks between meals, you can try having four or five small meals per day no more than two to three hours apart. The point of either of these alternatives is to maintain a steadier blood sugar level.

Supplements for hypoglycemia. The following supplements can be helpful in treating hypoglycemia:

- Vitamin B complex: 50 to 100 milligrams of all eleven B vitamins once per day with meals (when you are under stress, take two per day)

- Vitamin C: 1,000 milligrams twice per day with meals

- Chromium picolinate: 200 to 400 micrograms per day

- Glutamine: 500 milligrams a half-hour before lunch and a half-hour before dinner (this amino acid will help reduce sugar cravings)

- Magnesium: 200 to 600 milligrams per day

Vitamin B complex and vitamin C help to increase your resiliency to stress and limit blood sugar swings. The B vitamins also help regulate the metabolic processes that convert carbohydrates to sugar in your body. Chromium has a direct, stabilizing effect on your blood sugar level by facilitating the process by which insulin carries sugar to your cells. Magnesium has also been found to help stabilize blood sugar.

FOOD ALLERGIES

An allergic reaction occurs when your body tries to resist the intrusion of a foreign substance. For some people, certain foods affect the body like a foreign substance, causing not only classic allergic symptoms such as runny nose, mucus, and sneezing but a host of psychological or psychosomatic symptoms, including any of the following:

- anxiety or panic

- depression or mood swings

- dizziness

- irritability

- insomnia

- headaches

- confusion and disorientation

- fatigue

Such reactions occur in many individuals only when they eat an excessive amount of a particular food, eat a combination of offending foods, or have excessively low resistance due to a cold or infection. Others are so sensitive that even a small amount of the wrong food can cause debilitating symptoms. Often the subtler, psychological symptoms have a delayed onset, making it difficult to make the connection between food and symptom.

In our culture, the two most common foods causing allergic reactions are milk or dairy products and wheat. It is *casein* in milk and *gluten* in wheat (both are types of proteins) that tend to cause problems. Other foods that can trigger an allergic response include alcohol, chocolate, citrus fruits, corn, eggs, garlic, peanuts, yeast, shellfish, soy products, and tomatoes. One of the most telling signs of a food allergy is craving. You tend to crave the very foods to which you are allergic. While chocolate is the most flagrant example of this, you might also take pause if you find yourself tending to crave bread (wheat), corn chips (corn), dairy products, or another specific type of food. Many people go for years without recognizing that the very foods they crave the most have a subtle but toxic effect on their mood and well-being.

How can you find out whether food allergies are aggravating your problems with anxiety? There are clinical tests you can obtain from a nutritionally oriented doctor. Among formal clinical tests for food allergies, the *radioallergosorbent test* (RAST) and the *enzyme-linked immunosorbent assay* (ELISA) are probably the most reliable. These are blood tests that measure the number of antibodies you produce in reaction to a wide range of foods. Elevated numbers of antibodies in your blood after you've been exposed to a specific food indicate that you are allergic to that food. Such tests provide a detailed profile of all of the foods to which you're allergic and can be a very helpful diagnostic tool.

There are also nonscientific, and thus less conclusive, tests you can conduct on your own. The *elimination test* is one of these. If you want to determine whether you are allergic to wheat, simply eliminate all products containing wheat from your diet for two weeks and notice whether you feel better. Then, at the end of the two weeks, eat a large amount of wheat and carefully monitor any symptoms that appear over the next twenty-four hours. After testing wheat, you might want to test milk and milk products. It's important to experiment with only one potentially allergic type of food at a time so that you don't confound your results. Another nonscientific way to test for food allergies is to take your pulse after eating a meal. If it's elevated by more than ten beats per minute above your normal rate, it may be that you ate something you're allergic to.

The good news is that you probably do not have to permanently abstain from a food to which you are allergic. After a period of several months away from a food, you may be able to eat it again occasionally without adverse effects. For example, instead of having bread at almost every meal, you'll find that you feel better having it only a couple times per week.

Food allergies can definitely be a contributing factor to excessive anxiety and mood swings for certain people. If you suspect this to be a problem, your best course of action is to consult a physician or naturopath qualified to diagnose food allergies.

Nurturing Wellness with a Natural Diet

Eating a diet rich in whole, natural foods is an important key to maintaining overall wellness and can help limit your propensity for anxiety. As a general rule, the less processed your food, the better it is. Fresh, raw vegetables are more conducive to health than their cooked, frozen, or canned counterparts. You will glean more energy from an apple than a bag of buttered popcorn. Try to eat whole, unprocessed foods as often as possible. Whole foods include fresh fruits and vegetables, whole grains, unrefined cereals, beans, nuts, fresh fish, and free-range poultry. It's also important to eat a variety of foods so that you satisfy the full range of your body's needs. Your regular menu should include complex carbohydrates, such as vegetables and whole grains; fats, such as oils and nuts; and proteins, such as poultry, cold-water fish (salmon, for example), eggs, and soy products.

WHY LIMIT PROCESSED FOODS?

The nutrient content of processed food is compromised in two ways. First, the food is fragmented at a cellular level. For example, in the process of making white flour, the bran and germ of the wheat is split off, leaving only the pulp. Twenty different nutrients are removed in this process. When the flour is subsequently "enriched," only four nutrients are returned. Second, processed food contains additives and preservatives that are already partial or fragmented. These further reduce the nutritive value of food and, if eaten in large quantities, may pose serious health risks.

NATURAL FOODS ARE NO LONGER NATURAL CHOICES

Although no one can maintain a perfect diet all the time, it's important to strive for good nutrition whenever possible. This means appreciating your full range of food choices and being able to make informed decisions about which are the best ones. If you're in the mood for something sweet, make a fruit salad instead of reaching for a candy bar. Instead of having a bag of potato chips when you watch a rental movie, have a few carrot sticks with natural almond butter. For many of us, this means not going for the first food that comes to mind when we're craving sugar or just want to munch on something. It's ironic that natural foods are no longer "natural" choices, but an affinity for wholesome, healthy foods can be cultivated. If your diet routinely includes junk food, it might be a challenge at first, but changing to a more natural diet can have far-reaching benefits for your physical, emotional, and even spiritual health. What follows are some suggestions for upgrading your diet to one that promotes wellness—as well as greater calmness.

Eat more complex carbohydrates. Fresh fruits and vegetables, whole grains, whole-grain bread, and legumes are all rich sources of complex carbohydrates. These complex carbohydrate foods offer fiber, vitamins, minerals, and nutrients that can provide a measure of protection against chronic illnesses like diabetes, cancer, and heart disease.

Carbohydrates also seem to function as edible tranquilizers. They can increase the absorption of *tryptophan,* an amino acid that stimulates serotonin production in the brain. Serotonin generally has a calming effect.

Increase fiber in your diet. Evidence continues to mount that dietary fiber (including cellulose, gums, pectin, and lignin) is an essential component of a healthy diet. Fiber helps reduce constipation by increasing stool bulk and water absorption, controls blood sugar and blood lipids by binding nutrients, and decreases stool transit time, thus reducing the risk of colon cancer and other intestinal diseases. Even though the recommended daily intake of dietary fiber is twenty-five to forty grams, the average American consumes only five to ten grams a day. You can supplement your fiber intake by increasing your use of legumes and bran products or by adding bran to homemade foods. Also, you may want to have raw vegetables or a salad to accompany both lunch and dinner. Raw fruits are preferable between meals, since for many people it is difficult to digest fruit and proteins together. A certain amount of fiber is necessary, but too much (for example, a diet consisting solely of raw vegetables and whole grains) can stress the intestinal tract and cause bloating, so plan to increase your fiber gradually.

If you eat red meat, choose free-range, antibiotic-free beef. Free-range, antibiotic-free beef is a good source of protein and is high in *carnitine,* which boosts fat burning, energy, and mental acuity. It also gives your brain a degree of protection from stress.

Eat a variety of foods. Variety is the spice of life—and the foundation of a good diet. Just as a variety of experiences and relationships constitutes your life, a variety of foods should make up your diet. You need over forty nutrients for optimum health. These are classified as *macronutrients* (proteins, carbohydrates, and fats) and *micronutrients* (vitamins and minerals). You need the former in larger quantities and the latter in smaller amounts. Eating a variety of foods is essential for satisfying these needs.

You may have grappled with how you can get enough carbohydrates and protein and still keep the fat in your diet low. This can be done by selecting low-fat meat and dairy products whenever possible. Using beans and legumes liberally will help keep protein up and fat down. Informed food preparation can also help. The skin on a chicken breast has five grams of fat, so you should remove it. Bake, broil, or barbecue food to reduce fat.

Choose organic whenever possible. Organic foods are those fruits, vegetables, and grains that are grown with natural fertilizers and are not sprayed with pesticides or fungicides. Residues of these substances may be present in any fruit or vegetable not labeled organic. Meat and poultry in most stores is likely to contain steroid and antibiotic residues unless it's labeled organic or, in the case of chicken, free-range. In response to consumer demand, some supermarkets offer produce guaranteed to have little or no pesticide residue. Most health food stores also offer organic produce.

If organic vegetables and fruits are unavailable in your area, here are a few tips for minimizing your exposure to chemicals that may be on conventionally grown food:

- Wash all fruits and vegetables thoroughly before eating them.

- Remove the outer layers of head lettuce, cabbage, and other greens.

- Peel waxed produce such as apples or cucumbers.

- Avoid cooking with orange, lemon, or lime rind unless you obtain it from pesticide-free fruit.

If you drink, drink in moderation. As a tool for reducing stress, alcohol has the bothersome side effect of reducing reality as well. Although some research indicates that a drink a day will increase longevity, reliance on alcohol to deal with daily life is downright dangerous and sure to lead to addiction. Alcoholic beverages are high in calories and low in nutrients. In excess, alcohol depletes B vitamins, alters blood sugar, elevates blood pressure, and disrupts relationships. If you drink, limit yourself to one drink daily.

Eat more vegetables. Let's start with what you know: vegetables are an excellent source of vitamins, minerals, and fiber. Now for the surprising news: they can also be delectable. Unfortunately, in an era in which the standard diet is glutted with sweets, soda pop, and snack foods, vegetables have become a dietary casualty. Yet this dislike is likely to have been acquired (most babies like vegetable baby foods) and can be unlearned.

Retraining your palate to enjoy vegetables may not be as tough as you think. As you start to remove unhealthful foods from your diet, you'll probably discover how yummy vegetables can be when they are fresh and creatively prepared. Their natural flavors seem to come out best when they are lightly steamed. It's a good idea to eat both raw and cooked vegetables daily. A salad consisting of different kinds of lettuce, cucumbers, radishes, carrots, onions, and tomatoes is a good accompaniment to lunch or dinner. Cooked broccoli, spinach, asparagus, string beans, or greens such as kale, chard, or bok choy go well with fish and rice for dinner. Cruciferous vegetables (cabbage, broccoli, kale, collards, mustard greens, brussels sprouts) are better eaten cooked. These vegetables have several benefits, including protection against colon cancer. If your energy is low, you will likely feel better after eating a mixture of lightly steamed vegetables, along with whole grain rice and tofu for balance . . . and you just might enjoy it too.

Eat the right kinds of fat. It's not so much the quantity of fat we consume as the quality that matters. Eating the right fatty acids and having the right balance of them is necessary to make healthy cell membranes and regulate inflammatory responses. The right fats also help our bodies deal with stress. About 25 to 30 percent of the day's calorie intake should consist of healthy fats.

The balance between *omega-3, omega-6,* and *omega-9* fatty acids is critically important. The typical American diet contains plenty of omega-6 and omega-9 fatty acids but is deficient in omega-3 fatty acids. Omega-3 fatty acids can be found in flax-seed oil, pumpkin seed oil, hemp oil, olive oil, canola oil, walnuts, and fresh fish, especially salmon and sardines. One fatty acid in particular, *DHA,* an omega-3 fatty acid found in fish and fish oil capsules, is important for neurological and brain health.

Omega-3 fatty acids can also be found in natural animal and dairy fats, including cultured butter; organically raised, grass-fed sheep and beef; and in free-running poultry as well as in the egg yolks from this poultry. However, nutrition experts disagree about the role of animal fats in a healthy diet. Some experts feel that the saturated fats found in animal products are unhealthy and should be avoided. Others feel that saturated fats, in moderation and derived from the right sources, can be good for the body. If you choose to eat animal and dairy foods, buy organic products that are free of pesticides, antibiotics, and growth hormones.

As you shift your focus to healthy fats, you will want to reduce your consumption of polyunsaturated vegetable oils such as safflower, sunflower, sesame, corn, and soy oil. It is best to completely avoid *trans fats,* which are found in margarine, some potato and tortilla chips, most candy and cookies, many deep-fried foods, and all products containing partially hydrogenated oils. Read labels on processed foods and avoid items that contain partially hydrogenated oils.

Chew (really chew) your food. Think for a moment not about what you eat but how you eat it. If you eat too fast, or do not adequately chew your food, you'll miss a lot of the nutrient content as well as cause yourself indigestion. Digestion begins when you chew your food. If your food is not properly predigested in your mouth, much of it will not get adequately digested in your stomach. When this partially digested food passes on through your intestines, it's likely to ferment and cause bloating, cramps, and gas. In addition, you'll get only a limited amount of your food's potential nutrition, which can possibly lead to subtle forms of undernourishment.

To ensure you get the full value of your food, give yourself time to eat, and chew each mouthful of solid food at least fifteen to twenty times. If, after doing this, you still feel bloated or have problems with indigestion, you may want to talk to your doctor or health practitioner about taking digestive enzymes (available at health food stores) with or after each meal. If you properly digest your food, you should feel satisfied and comfortable after a meal rather than dull or lethargic.

Attain or maintain a healthy weight. Although we are awash in diet schemes that promise speedy results, the best weight control program is a lifelong plan of consistent, sensible eating. Diets just don't work. Research indicates that "yo-yo dieting" damages health and makes each successive weight-loss effort even harder. Diets are just a temporary fix, while true weight control is an issue that must be addressed throughout our lives.

Below are some pointers for reaching a healthy weight. Regular aerobic exercise will help too, by raising your metabolic rate.

- Eat slowly. Take small bites and give yourself time to delight in the color, taste, and texture of the food. Remember that it takes twenty minutes for your *hypothalamus* (your "appestat") to register satiety or a sense of fullness.

- Concentrate on eating. Don't read or watch TV while you're eating. Enjoy eating as a primary activity so you can be aware of flavors, colors, and portion size.

- Eat regularly. Studies show that people who eat three to four meals daily tend to control their weight successfully. This may be because they do not get excessively hungry and overeat or snack between meals. Studies also indicate that those who eat breakfast consume fewer daily calories.

- When you're anxious, use the relaxation techniques suggested in chapter 1, go to a movie, or do physical exercise, preferably aerobic.

- When you're bored, allow yourself a pleasurable activity such as going for a walk, calling a friend, or engaging in a hobby.

- When you're angry, write a letter to the person you're angry with (but don't send it), or go jogging or do some gardening. If you must chew something, choose a carrot or sugarless gum.

- When you're tired, go to bed or take a hot bath. You may be surprised to find that a walk or a bike ride reenergizes you.

Water, water (should be) everywhere. You should try to drink six to eight eight-ounce glasses of purified water per day. Why? A primary reason is that water helps your kidneys. The main function of your kidneys is to filter out all kinds of toxic waste products of bodily metabolism as well as chemical and environmental pollutants from the outside. For your kidneys to operate properly, you need to drink plentiful amounts of water to help wash away waste. You especially need to drink ample water if you live in a hot environment, eat a lot of protein, drink alcohol or coffee, take medications, are running a fever, or have urinary problems.

The purity of the water you drink is important. Most water purification plants focus on disinfection, largely ignoring chemical contamination from industrial or agricultural wastes that find their way into groundwater. Disinfection is often accomplished through chlorination, which poses additional hazards. Chlorine is a poisonous gas that can yield toxic by-products, *trihalomethanes,* which are known to cause cancer and birth defects. Chlorine also displaces iodine, interfering with the production of thyroid hormone. This may lead to *hypothyroidism,* which can cause, among other symptoms, weight gain and depression. For all of these reasons, the tap is probably not the best source of water.

You can buy bottled water or attach a water purification system to your tap. If you buy bottled water, make sure the label includes a detailed analysis of its contents. Some spring waters may come from sources that have been affected by contaminated groundwater. The two most common types of water purification systems are activated carbon filters and reverse osmosis systems. Both filter out chlorine and toxic organic molecules; however, reverse osmosis systems will also filter out toxic metals. The downside of reverse osmosis systems is that they waste a lot of water. Filters in activated carbon filter systems must be periodically replaced. Either system is a vast improvement over plain tap water and certainly more convenient and cost-effective than continually purchasing bottled water.

Cut back on milk and milk products if you are lactose intolerant or are allergic to dairy products. Let's consider a few facts about milk and milk products. Lactose is part of the carbohydrate component of milk. Like many people, you may be lactose intolerant, which means that your stomach does not make the digestive enzyme *lactase*. Lactase is needed to digest lactose. As a result, when you drink milk, you may experience bloating, excessive gas, and general intestinal distress.

The protein in milk (casein) can produce an allergic response, most frequently in the form of mucus. It is common for milk and dairy products to aggravate chronic allergic conditions such as asthma, bronchitis, and sinusitis. Milk is also known to aggravate autoimmune conditions such as rheumatoid arthritis and lupus.

Much of the commercial milk you drink contains residues of drugs and hormones used to increase the productivity of cows. Homogenization of milk removes bacteria but not the hormone residues. Raw milk from a certified dairy is likely to lack hormones, but it may contain bacteria.

Not a rosy picture, is it? Now for some good news: If you choose to drink less milk, there are substitutes, like soy or rice milk, available to you. Most people learn to enjoy them just as much as milk. You can find both of them in health food stores and even some conventional supermarkets. You may also want to try soy-based cheeses. If you eat milk-based cheeses, opt for the low-fat or nonfat varieties.

Increase the amount of protein relative to the amount of carbohydrate in your diet. Until a few years ago, many nutritionists advocated allocating as much as 70 percent of total daily calories to complex carbohydrates. The prevailing idea was that too much fat promoted cardiovascular disease and too much protein led to excessive acidity and toxicity in the body. The ideal diet was thought to consist of 15 to 20 percent fat, 15 to 20 percent protein, and the rest carbohydrates. In the past few years, however, evidence has mounted against the idea of eating high quantities of carbohydrates, especially by themselves.

Carbohydrates are used by the body to produce glucose, the form of sugar the body and brain use for fuel. In order to transport glucose to the cells, your pancreas secretes insulin. Eating high levels of carbohydrates means your body produces higher levels of insulin, and too much insulin has an adverse effect on some of the body's most basic hormonal and neuroendocrine systems.

Eating large amounts of cereals, breads, pastas—or even grains such as rice or vegetables such as carrots, corn, and potatoes—can raise your insulin levels to the point that other basic systems are thrown out of balance. The answer is not to eliminate carbohydrates but to reduce them in proportion to the amounts of protein and fat you consume, without increasing the total number of calories in your diet. By doing this, you'll not end up eating a diet that is too high in fat or protein. Instead, you'll continue to eat fats and protein in moderation while decreasing the amount of carbohydrate you have at each meal relative to the amounts of fat and protein. The optimal ratio may be 25 to 30 percent protein, 25 to 30 percent fat (unless you are on a low-fat diet to reduce risk of heart disease), and 40 to 50 percent carbohydrate, with vegetable sources of protein and fat preferable to animal.

In his 1995 book *The Zone,* Barry Sears presents considerable research supporting the value of reducing the proportion of carbohydrate to protein and fat. Some anxiety sufferers have reported that increasing protein relative to carbohydrate at each meal reduces anxiety. This isn't surprising, because anxiety and mood disorders often involve deficiencies in neurotransmitters, especially serotonin. The body has no way to make neuro-transmitters (and serotonin in particular) without a steady supply of amino acids, which are derived from protein. Whether or not you decide to adopt a 40:30:30 diet, it's a good idea to have some protein (preferably in the form of fish, organic poultry, tofu, tempeh, eggs, unprocessed cheese, or beans and grains) at every meal. On the other hand, aim not to exceed 30 percent protein, especially in the form of meat, chicken, or fish, as this may tend to make your body overly acidic.

If you eat out, do it in a healthy way. The unremitting pace of modern life is a boon for the food service industry. For many of us, eating out is less a treat than a necessity if we want to stick to our busy schedules. The problem is that most restaurant food, even at its best, packs too many calories, too much saturated fat, and too much salt. Also, much of the food you eat at a restaurant doesn't have the freshness you would opt for if you were prepar-ing it yourself. In general, eating out regularly is not a habit that benefits your health, but if you can't avoid it, here are a few tips for making it as healthy as possible:

- Avoid fast food or junk food concessions.

- Whenever possible, eat out at natural food or health food restaurants that use whole, preferably organic, foods.

- If natural food restaurants are unavailable, go to high-quality seafood restaurants and order fresh fish, preferably broiled or baked. Accompany the fish with fresh vegetables, potatoes or rice, and a green salad. On the salad, avoid creamy or dairy-based dressings.

- As a third choice, try a high-quality Chinese or Japa-nese restaurant, and have a meal of rice, vegetables, and fresh fish or tofu. In Chinese restaurants, request that your meals be prepared without MSG (mono-sodium glutamate), a flavor enhancer to which many people are allergic.

- As a general rule, avoid eating the rolls or bread that often come with a meal, and don't order cream-based soups such as clam chowder.

- Stick with simple entrées such as chicken or whitefish without elaborate sauces or toppings.

- Try to resist high-fat desserts.

- Don't hesitate to ask to have food prepared according to your needs. You're paying for it, so you have every right to expect your meal to be prepared to your liking.

- Learn to enjoy the subtle tastes of simple foods. This becomes easy and desirable after a while when you omit rich, high-fat, and sugary foods.

Let Change Happen Naturally

Whew! You just got quite a laundry list of suggestions for upgrading your diet. If you're unaccustomed to thinking about what you eat, it can seem overwhelming. Keep in mind, though, that you don't have to implement all these changes at once. Try decreasing your caffeine and sugar consumption first, since these are most closely linked to your anxiety. Beyond that, let your diet change naturally, at your own pace. Make a new change when you feel you are ready for it. You're more likely to stick to those dietary changes that you implement in the spirit of healing and self-love than to those you force upon yourself.

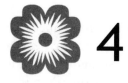 4

Thinking Calm

Imagine two people waiting in an airport terminal for a plane that was supposed to take off a half hour ago. One person thinks, *Just my luck! Now I'm stuck here with nothing to do for who knows how long. I have so much to do when I get home, and this is going to throw my schedule completely off. Ugh, I'm going to go crazy if I have to wait much longer!* Not surprisingly, she feels jumpy, anxious, and irritated. The other thinks, *Since I have to stay here, I might as well make the best of it. I'll catch up on my reading and maybe write a letter to my friend whom I just visited, or I can do some abdominal breathing and listen to music on my Walkman.* She feels peaceful, calm, and in control.

This illustrates how what we think about a given event can determine our feelings about it more than the event itself. Thoughts can seem so reflexive that it's easy to believe that it's the situation that "makes" us feel a certain way, rather than what we tell ourselves about it. The truth is that it's mainly what we say to ourselves in response to any particular situation that determines our mood and feelings. In short, you are largely responsible for how you feel (barring physical stresses, such as illness).

This is a profound and very important truth—one that sometimes takes a long time to fully grasp. It's often much easier to blame the way you feel on something or someone outside yourself than to take responsibility for your reactions. Yet it is through your willingness to accept that responsibility that you begin to take charge and have mastery over your life. The realization that you are mostly responsible for how you feel is empowering once you fully accept it. It's one of the most important keys to living a happier, more effective, and anxiety-free life.

In this chapter we'll look at the fearful thoughts that fuel panic attacks, phobias, and worry. If you suffer from any of these forms of anxiety, you know that when you feel their symptoms, your thoughts take on a distinctively catastrophic bent. Thoughts like *I'm going to go crazy* often surface when you feel the first stirrings of panic. What-if statements are a common denominator of all forms of worry: *What if I have cancer?* or *What if they don't like me?* Anxiety surrounding a phobic situation is often intensified by thoughts that predict dire (and unlikely) outcomes, such as *I have to give a talk at work. What if I panic? Everyone will think I'm crazy and I'll never be taken seriously again. I'd have to quit my job.* Being able to replace these catastrophic thoughts with more realistic ones is a key skill in anxiety control. The exercises in this chapter are designed to help you master this skill.

About Panic Attacks

Panic is the most extreme form of anxiety. When you have a panic attack, you experience a surge of mounting physiological arousal that culminates in peak-intensity anxiety symptoms. If "normal" anxiety is a campfire, panic is an inferno. Common physical symptoms include heart palpitations, tightening in the chest, shortness of breath, dizziness, faintness, sweating, nausea, trembling, shaking, and tingling in the hands and feet. Fears of "going crazy," having a heart attack, or dying often spring up around these physical sensations. Feelings of unreality and an intense desire to flee are also typical. Panic can occur spontaneously or in response to encountering a phobic situation.

Your very first panic attack can have a traumatic impact, leaving you feeling terrified, helpless, and anxious about the possibility of future episodes. Unfortunately, in some cases, panic does repeatedly recur. Why some people have a panic attack only once—or perhaps once every few years—while others develop a chronic condition with several attacks per week is still not well understood.

The good news is that you can learn to cope with panic attacks so that they will no longer have the power to frighten you. There are both long- and short-term interventions that can help you diminish the intensity and frequency of panic attacks. Long-term interventions include changes in your lifestyle described elsewhere in this book. Particularly important are regular practice of deep relaxation (chapter 1), maintaining an exercise routine (chapter 2), eliminating caffeine and sugar from your diet (chapter 3), and simplifying your life (chapter 9). Short-term strategies are the focus of this chapter and include challenging fearful self-talk and using coping statements.

PANIC ATTACKS ARE NOT DANGEROUS

Anyone who has panic attacks knows that it's impossible to exaggerate the feelings of terror that they trigger. When you're in the grip of an attack, the anxiety is so great that it can feel like a desperate, even deadly, situation is at hand. Fears of death or serious harm may seem only logical. Yet, the truth about panic attacks is that they are not dangerous. They cannot cause a heart attack, stroke, suffocation, sudden death, or any other physical calamity. They cannot cause you to "go crazy" or "lose it." These fears arise because, despite the absence of any true threat, your body sends clear danger signals to your mind. Your mind then conjures up a danger to match your bodily symptoms. The following symptoms and fearful thoughts tend to go hand in hand.

Symptom	Fearful Thought
heart palpitations	*I'm going to have a heart attack or I'm going to die.*
choking sensation	*I'm going to stop breathing and suffocate.*
dizzy sensation	*I'm going to pass out.*
feeling disoriented or "not all there"	*I'm going crazy.*
"rubbery" legs	*I'm going to fall or I won't be able to walk.*
overall intensity of your physical reaction	*I'm going to completely lose control of myself or I'm going crazy.*

The moment you tell yourself that danger is at hand, you multiply the intensity of your fear, which in turn makes your bodily symptoms worse, which creates still more fear, and you get caught in an upward spiral of mounting panic. This upward spiral can be avoided if you fully accept that what your body is going through is not dangerous. All of the above dangers are illusory, a product of your imagination when you're undergoing the intense reactions that constitute panic. There is simply no basis for any of these fears in reality, and reminding yourself of this is the first step in overcoming panic. Let's examine each fear one by one.

A panic attack cannot cause heart failure or cardiac arrest. Rapid heartbeat and palpitations during a panic attack can be frightening sensations, but they're not dangerous. Your heart is made up of very strong and dense muscle fibers and can withstand a lot more than you might think. A healthy heart can beat 200 beats per minute for many hours without sustaining any damage. So, if your heart begins to race, just allow it to do so, trusting that no harm can come of it and that your heart will eventually calm down. Panic attacks are not hazardous to your heart.

A panic attack will not cause you to stop breathing or suffocate. It is common during panic to feel your chest close down and your breathing become restricted. This might lead you to suddenly fear that you're going to suffocate. Under stress, your neck and chest muscles are tightening and reducing your respiratory capacity. Be assured that there is nothing wrong with your breathing passage or lungs, and that the tightening sensations will pass. Your brain has a built-in reflex mechanism that will eventually force you to breathe if you're not getting enough oxygen. At a certain point you'll feel a strong reflex to take in more air. The same thing will happen in a panic attack if you're not getting enough oxygen. You'll automatically gasp and take a deep breath long before reaching the point where you could pass out from a lack of oxygen. (And even if you did pass out, you would immediately start breathing!) In sum, choking and sensations of constriction during panic, however unpleasant, are not dangerous.

A panic attack cannot cause you to faint. The sensation of light-headedness you may feel with the onset of panic can evoke a fear of fainting. What is happening is that the blood circulation to your brain is slightly reduced, most likely because you are breathing more rapidly. This is not dangerous and can be relieved by deliberately breathing slowly and regularly from your abdomen, preferably through your nose. This feeling can also be helped by walking around as soon as you have the opportunity. Let the feelings of light-headedness rise and subside without fighting them.

A panic attack cannot cause you to lose your balance. You may feel quite dizzy when panic comes on. It may be that tension is affecting the semicircular canal system in your inner ear, which regulates your balance. For a few moments you may feel dizzy, or it may even seem that things around you are spinning. Invariably this sensation will pass. It isn't dangerous, and it's very unlikely to be so strong that you'll actually lose your balance. If sensations of pronounced dizziness persist for more than a few minutes, you may want to consult a doctor (preferably an *otolaryngologist,* an ear, nose, and throat doctor) to check if infection, allergies, or other disturbances might be affecting your inner ear.

You won't fall when you feel weak in the knees during a panic attack. The adrenaline released during a panic attack can dilate the blood vessels in your legs, causing blood to accumulate in your leg muscles and not fully circulate. This can produce a sensation of weakness or "jelly legs," to which you may respond with the fear that you won't be able to walk. Be assured that this sensation is just that: a sensation, and that your legs are as strong and able to carry you as ever. They won't give way! Just allow these trembling, weak sensations to pass and give your legs the chance to carry you where you need to go.

You can't "go crazy" during a panic attack. Reduced blood flow to your brain during a panic attack is due to arterial constriction, a normal consequence of rapid breathing. This can result in sensations of disorientation and a feeling of unreality that can be frightening. If this sensation comes on, remind yourself that it's simply due to a slight and temporary reduction of arterial circulation in your brain and does not have anything to do with "going crazy," no matter how eerie or strange it may feel. No one has ever "gone crazy" from a panic attack, even though the fear of doing so is common. As bad as they feel, sensations of unreality will eventually pass and are completely harmless.

It may be helpful to know that people do not "go crazy" in a sudden or spontaneous way. Mental disorders involving behaviors that are labeled "crazy" (such as schizophrenia or manic-depressive psychosis) develop very gradually over a period of years and do not arise from panic attacks. No one has ever started to hallucinate or hear voices during a panic attack (except in rare instances where panic was induced by an overdose of a recreational drug such as LSD or cocaine). In short, a panic attack cannot result in your "going crazy," no matter how disturbing or unpleasant your symptoms feel.

A panic attack cannot cause you to "lose control" of yourself. Because of the intense reactions your body goes through during panic, it's easy to imagine that you could "completely lose it."

But what does *completely losing it* mean? Becoming completely paralyzed? Acting out uncontrollably or running amok? There is no recorded instance of this happening. If anything, during panic your senses and awareness are heightened with respect to a single goal: escape. Running away or trying to run away are the only ways in which you would be likely to "act out" while panicking. Complete loss of control during panic attacks is simply a myth.

The Panic Sequence

A panic attack is the result of a sequence of events involving unpleasant body symptoms and catastrophic thoughts. Those who are prone to panic tend to interpret body symptoms such as heart palpitations or dizziness as dangerous or potentially catastrophic. The panic sequence is illustrated below.

Initial Stimulus
(for example, underbreathing, being stuck in traffic)

↓

Worry
(for example, *What if I start to panic?*)

↓

Early Physiological Arousal
(mild symptoms, for example, "butterflies," increased heart rate, sweaty palms, slight dizziness)

↓

Catastrophic Thoughts
(for example, *I'm having a heart attack* or
I'm going to go crazy)

↓

Heightened Physiological Arousal

THE INITIAL STIMULUS

The initial stimulus is the event or situation that sparks the panic cycle. An initial stimulus can be an external event, such as confronting a situation in which you panicked before, or an internal one, like a rapid heartbeat or underbreathing. Whether or not you're aware of the stimulus, you start to worry.

WORRY

Your worry thoughts may be so instantaneous that they seem automatic. Worry thoughts might include:

What if I panic here again?

I'm starting to get dizzy—am I going to lose it again?

Something feels off—I need to get out of here!

Uh-oh—here it comes.

Worry thoughts give way to the next phase in the panic sequence: physiological arousal.

PHYSIOLOGICAL AROUSAL

Your body is programmed to interpret any potential danger as a threat that you need to fight or flee. This is why within seconds of the worry thoughts, physiological symptoms such as rapid heartbeat, increasing respiration, muscle tension, and perspiration begin or intensify. Psychologically, you feel uneasy. If you perceive these body symptoms as dangerous, you will trigger an alarm reaction in your body that's likely to lead to panic. All mammals have this built-in alarm reaction so that they can fight or flee predators. When it's activated, the following physiological reactions occur:

- Your heart rate quickly increases to provide blood to the large muscles so that you can run or do battle.

- Your rate of breathing increases to provide energy for sudden, rapid movement (what you may feel is tightness in your chest).

- The blood supply to your brain is slightly decreased and redirected toward your large muscles (what you may feel is sensations of dizziness, confusion, or unreality).

- The blood flow to your extremities is diminished to reduce bleeding if you're injured (what you may feel is cold hands or feet at the same time that you feel flushed).

- Sweating is triggered so that your skin will be hard for a predator to grasp.

- Digestion is slowed (what you may feel is cramping and nausea).

While these symptoms are harmless, you may respond to them by entering into the next phase of the panic sequence: thinking catastrophic thoughts.

CATASTROPHIC THOUGHTS

Catastrophic thoughts signal your body to ratchet up its fight-or-flight preparation even more.

Examples of catastrophic thoughts might include:

I'm going to have a heart attack if I don't get out of here.

I'll pass out before I can get off the freeway (or through the stoplight).

I'll start to stammer and make a fool of myself.

I'm going to go crazy!

This is the end—I'm dying!

These thoughts ultimately lead to very heightened physio-logical arousal, which is the final phase in the panic sequence.

HEIGHTENED PHYSIOLOGICAL AROUSAL

When your body gets the message that you're in imminent danger (even though in actuality you're not), it releases massive amounts of adrenaline, which in turn triggers more catastrophic thoughts, which in turn propels the physical symptoms to even greater levels of intensity. This culminates in a full-blown panic attack.

Cutting Short the Panic Sequence

Freeing yourself from panic means interrupting the panic sequence when it's still in its early stages. To be able to do this, you must recognize and remind yourself that panic symptoms do not lead to anything catastrophic. It's worth repeating: *Panic attacks are not dangerous*. Yes, they can be uncomfortable, but they cannot cause lasting physical damage or precipitate any dev-astating physical or psychological event. If you learn to replace catastrophic thoughts like *I'm going to lose control of myself and go crazy* with realistic ones such as *This is only panic. It can't hurt me*, you will be better able to cut short the panic sequence. The following exercise is designed to help you challenge and change the catastrophic thoughts that fuel the panic sequence.

Changing Catastrophic Thoughts to Realistic Ones

Replacing your catastrophic thoughts with realistic ones is a three-part process. First you have to recognize your particular catastrophic thoughts, then you have to question their validity, and lastly you have to replace them with more realistic thoughts.

Exercise: Changing Catastrophic Thoughts Associated with Panic

To begin this exercise, take a blank piece of paper and draw a line vertically down the center, creating two columns. Label the left-hand column *Catastrophic Thoughts* and the right-hand column *Realistic Thoughts*.

Step 1: Identify your catastrophic thoughts in response to the physical sensations of panic.

Think about what goes through your mind when panic symptoms arise. What kind of thoughts make the most trouble for you when you have a severe anxiety or panic episode? If you're unclear about what your catastrophic thoughts are, monitor yourself over the next two weeks, watching for the catastrophic thoughts that precede times when you feel anxious or panicky. Take time after your anxiety subsides to reflect on the fearful, scary thoughts that went through your mind. A list of common catastrophic thoughts appears below. You may recognize some of the thoughts on the list as your own. Most likely some of your catastrophic thoughts are not on the list, however, and it's important that you identify your own particular thoughts as well. Write your catastrophic thoughts under *Catastrophic Thoughts* on the worksheet.

I'm going to die.
I'm going insane.
I'm losing control.
This will never end.
I'm really scared.
I'm having a heart attack.
I'm going to pass out.
I'm going to make a scene.
I've got to get out of here.
I'm going to act foolish.
People will think I'm crazy.
I'll always be this way.
I don't understand what's happening to me.
Something is really physically wrong with me.
I'm losing my mind.

I'll choke to death.
I don't know what people will think.
I'm going blind.
I'll hurt someone.
I'm going to have a stroke.
I'm going to scream.
I'm going to babble or talk funny.
I'm going to throw up.
I won't be able to breathe.
Something terrible will happen.

Step 2: Ask yourself, *How realistic is this thought?*

Look at each catastrophic thought objectively and ask yourself how realistic it is. Challenge the validity of your catastrophic thoughts using the following questions:

- How many times in the past did the catastrophe I imagine actually occur?

- What has usually happened under similar circumstances, that is, when I've panicked, in the past?

- What are the objective medical facts (if your catastrophic thought relates to some bodily danger, such as a heart attack or suffocation)? Refer to the earlier section *Panic Attacks Are Not Dangerous.*

Step 3: Replace your catastrophic thoughts in response to the physical sensations of panic with more realistic ones.

Suppose you're scaring yourself with the catastrophic thought *I'm so dizzy I'm going to pass out!* In this step you formulate a more realistic thought based on the objective facts that you examined in step 2. Write it under *Realistic Thoughts* on the worksheet. Continuing with the above example, your new thought might be *I'm in the early stages of panic, and that's why I'm feeling dizzy. No one has ever fainted or passed out as a result of a panic attack. This will eventually pass and is not at all dangerous.*

First Fear and Second Fear

In *Hope and Help for Your Nerves and Peace from Nervous Suffering* (1978), Claire Weekes distinguishes between *first fear* and *second fear*. First fear comes with the initial symptoms of panic. When you feel the onset of symptoms like elevated heart rate, sweating, and dizziness, you're experiencing first fear. Fearful thoughts about these symptoms generate second fear. When you start telling yourself things like *I can't handle this, I've got to get out of here right now,* or *What if other people see this happening to me,* second fear takes hold and compounds your symptoms. While you can't do much about first fear, you can eliminate second fear by learning to flow with the rise and fall of your body's state of arousal rather than fighting or reacting fearfully. If you can keep second fear at bay, the physiological reaction will pass without you becoming so afraid of it. Much of the adrenaline that causes panic will be metabolized and reabsorbed by your body within five minutes. When this happens your physical symptoms will start to subside.

SECOND-FEAR STOPPER: COPING STATEMENTS

While first fear may occur randomly, second fear is a direct result of catastrophic self-talk. If you tell yourself that your symptoms are threatening and that you are on the brink of disaster, you'll scare yourself into a very high state of anxiety. Saying things like *I'm going to go crazy* or *I can't handle this anymore* will almost certainly bring about second fear. Conversely, saying reassuring things to yourself like *It's only anxiety—I'm not going to let it get to me, I've been through this before and it's not dangerous,* or *I can handle this until it passes* will likely deter second fear and reduce first fear.

Practice using any of the following coping statements to help you cultivate an attitude of accepting the body symptoms that occur during a panic attack. You may find it helpful to repeat a particular statement over and over the first minute or two, when you feel panic symptoms coming on. You may also want to do deep abdominal breathing in conjunction with repeating a coping statement. If one statement gets tiresome or seems to stop working, try another.

- *This feeling isn't comfortable or pleasant, but I can accept it.*

- *I can be anxious and still deal with this situation.*

- *I can handle these symptoms or sensations.*

- *This isn't an emergency. It's okay to think slowly about what I need to do.*

- *This isn't the worst thing that could happen.*

- *I'm going to go with this and wait for my anxiety to decrease.*

- *This is an opportunity for me to learn to cope with my fears.*

- *I'll just let my body do its thing. This will pass.*

- *I'll ride this through—I don't need to let this get to me.*

- *I deserve to feel okay right now.*

- *I can take all the time I need in order to let go and relax.*

- *There's no need to push myself. I can take as small a step forward as I choose.*

- *I've survived this before and I'll survive this time, too.*

- *I can do my coping strategies and allow this to pass.*

- *This anxiety won't hurt me, even if it doesn't feel good.*

- *This is just anxiety. I'm not going to let it get to me.*

- *Nothing serious is going to happen to me.*

- *Fighting and resisting this isn't going to help, so I'll just ride it through.*

- *These are just thoughts, not reality.*

- *I don't need these thoughts. I can choose to think differently.*

- *This isn't dangerous.*

- *So what.*

- *These sensations (feelings) are just a reminder to use my coping skills.*

- *These feelings will pass and I'll be okay.*

- *This is just adrenaline and it will pass in a few minutes.*

- *Nothing about these sensations or feelings is dangerous.*

- *Don't worry, be happy.* (Use this, if you like, to inject an element of lightness or humor).

While you are using coping statements to quell the early symptoms of panic, the best thing to do is to begin abdominal breathing (see next section). If you have frequent panic attacks, it's a good idea to write your favorite coping statements on a 3-by-5 card and carry it in your purse or wallet. Bring the card out and read it when you feel panic symptoms first coming on. If you have a problem with driving, tape a card with coping statements to your dashboard. Remember to combine the use of coping statements with abdominal breathing.

SECOND-FEAR STOPPER: ABDOMINAL BREATHING

Abdominal breathing by itself can stop panic and foster a deep sense of relaxation. It is a simple yet powerful technique for disarming the physiological symptoms of anxiety. If you use it in the early stages of panic, it can stave off second fear and help dissipate the symptoms of first fear. For detailed instructions on abdominal breathing, see chapter 1.

CREATE A DIVERSION

While abdominal breathing and coping statements should be your first line of defense, any of the following diversion strategies can also be helpful during the onset of panic or for any occasion when you feel anxious.

- Talk to another person. This could be someone with you or someone you can call.

- Move around or engage in physical activity.

- Engage in a simple, repetitive activity. For example, count the money in your purse while waiting in line, or sing a song during a long elevator ride.

- Express angry feelings. Get angry at your anxiety —just don't vent anger on other people. Shout at it with statements like *You're not going to run my life!*

- Anchor yourself in your immediate environment. Focus on concrete objects in your surroundings; even touch them if that helps.

- Practice *thought-stopping*. Shout the word *stop* once or twice, or snap a rubber band against your wrist. This will help disrupt a chain of negative thoughts. Follow this with abdominal breathing or by repeating a coping statement. Take time after your anxiety subsides to reflect on fearful thoughts that went through your mind.

About Phobias and Worry

Phobias and chronic worry are perpetuated by three elements: sensitization, avoidance, and fearful, erroneous self-talk.

A phobia develops when you become *sensitized* to a particular situation, object, or event—that is, when anxiety becomes conditioned or associated with that situation, object, or event. If high anxiety suddenly arises one day when you happen to be flying, driving, or riding in an elevator, you may start feeling anxious every time you subsequently enter these situations. Becoming sensitized means that the mere presence—or even the mere thought—of a situation may be enough to trigger anxiety.

After sensitization occurs, you may start to avoid the situation. When you avoid something consistently, you have a phobia. *Avoidance* is a natural but ineffective coping method. It's understandable that you would want to stay away from the situation that aroused so much fear, but the problem is that avoidance prevents you from ever learning that you can handle the situation, and thereby bolsters the phobia. Remember the old joke about the patient who goes to the doctor and says, "It hurts when I move my arm," and the doctor says, "Then don't move your arm"? Such a doctor would also prescribe avoidance of the phobic situation or object.

This does not mean, however, that you should abruptly immerse yourself in a phobic situation. You want to face the situation through a series of incremental exposures, possibly with the help of another person. Confronting phobias should be done in a gradual and measured way. For more information on exposing yourself to a phobic situation, see chapter 4 of *Coping with Anxiety* (Bourne and Garano) or consult a therapist trained in treating phobias.

The third factor that perpetuates phobias, and also the major factor in worry, is erroneous, exaggerated self-talk. The more worry you experience about something you fear, the more likely you are to engage in erroneous self-talk connected with that fear. You may also have negative images about what could happen if you had to face what you fear, or about your worst fears coming true. Both the negative self-talk and negative images serve to perpetuate your fear, guaranteeing that you remain afraid. They also undermine your confidence that you could ever get over your fear. By getting past your unrealistic self-talk and negative images, you will be more likely to overcome your avoidance and confront whatever it is you fear.

OVERESTIMATION AND UNDERESTIMATION

Phobias and fears come in many forms, but the nature of the catastrophic self-talk that underlies them is always the same. Whether you are afraid of crossing bridges, developing a serious illness, speaking up in groups, or getting an injection, the types of erroneous thinking that perpetuate these fears are the same. There are two basic errors in fearful thinking: *overestimating* the likelihood of a danger or threat and *underestimating* your ability to cope with it.

When you overestimate the likelihood of a danger, you fixate on the worst imaginable scenario even though it is probably the least likely. Your thoughts typically begin with *What if*. For example, you may think things like *What if I have cancer?* or *What if I flunk the exam and have to drop out of school?*

Implicit in these thoughts is an underestimation of your ability to cope with the feared outcome. The underlying message conveyed by these what-if statements is that the feared outcome would spell unavoidable ruin. When you begin to challenge your catastrophic thoughts, you'll see that even if what you fear the most materialized, you would have a variety of coping strategies at your disposal. This means that you would have at least some measure of control over how the feared event affected your life. The following examples illustrate how overestimation and underestimation play out in various fears and how you can counter them with more realistic self-talk.

Example: Fear of Serious Illness

Catastrophic pattern of thought. *I have no energy and feel tired all the time. What if I have cancer and don't know it? If I were diagnosed with cancer, that would be the end. I couldn't take it. I'd be better off ending things quickly and killing myself.*

Identify the distorted thoughts. The distorted thoughts are *Because I have low energy and feel tired, I must have cancer* and *If I had cancer, I certainly couldn't cope.* In identifying distorted thoughts, first list all of your what-ifs about the situation, then change them to affirmative statements. For example, *What if my low energy and fatigue are signs of cancer?* would get changed to *Because I have low energy and fatigue, I have cancer.*

Question their validity. *What are the odds that low energy and fatigue mean that I have cancer? If the unlikely happened and I really was diagnosed with cancer, how terrible could that be? Would I actually go to pieces and not be able to continue living? Realistically, is it true that I would have no way of coping with the situation?* Note how the questions begin. In challenging the validity of your catastrophic thoughts, it's helpful to use questions like:

- *What are the odds?*

- *Realistically, how likely is that?*

- *How often has that happened in the past?*

- *If the worst did happen, is it really true that I'd not find any way to cope?*

Replace them with more realistic ones. *Symptoms of fatigue and low energy can be indicative of all kinds of physical and psychological conditions, including a low-grade virus, anemia, adrenal exhaustion or hypothyroidism, depression, and food allergies, just to name a few. There are many possible explanations for my condition, and I don't have any specific symptoms that would indicate cancer. So the odds of my fatigue and low energy indicating* *cancer are very low. Moreover, bad as a cancer diagnosis would be, it's unlikely that I would totally go to pieces. After an initial difficult adjustment to the fact, which might take days to weeks, I would begin to think about what I needed to do to deal with the situation. It would certainly be difficult, but I wouldn't be less equipped to handle it than anyone else. My doctor and I would plan the most effective possible treatment strategies. I would join a local cancer support group and draw lots of support from my friends and immediate family. I would supplement my treatment with alternative methods, such as visualization and dietary changes, which could aid recovery. In short, I would do everything possible to heal the condition.*

Example: Fear of Panicking While Speaking before an Audience

Catastrophic pattern of thought. *What if I start to panic while giving a talk to those people? What if they think I'm crazy? I'd never live it down.*

Identify the distorted thoughts. The distorted thoughts are *I would surely panic if I had to give a talk* and *Others would definitely think I was crazy, which would be devastating to me.*

Question their validity. *Realistically, how likely is it that I would panic while speaking? What are the odds, if I did panic, that people would be aware of what I was thinking and thus conclude that I was crazy? Suppose the unlikely happened and people really thought I was crazy because I panicked. How terrible would that be? Is it realistic to suppose I'd never live it down?*

Replace them with more realistic ones. *If I did start to panic, I could simply abbreviate what I wanted to say and sit back down. As people tend to be caught up in their own thoughts and preoccupations, no one would likely notice my difficulty or be upset that I'd cut my comments short. Even if people did detect signs of panic, like my face turning red or my voice trembling, the odds are very slim that they'd think I was crazy or weird. Would I think that of someone if the roles were reversed? It's much more* *likely that they'd express concern. And even in the rare instance that someone thought I was crazy or different because I panicked, I could explain to them that I sometimes have a fear of speaking in public. With all the publicity about anxiety disorders these days, they would likely understand. Being totally honest is one way I could handle the situation. And no matter what happened, I would forget about it after a while. It's just not true that I would never live it down. I've gotten over embarrassment before.*

Example: Fear of Losing Your Job

Catastrophic pattern of thought. *The economy has tightened in the last couple of years and layoffs are skyrocketing. What if I lose my job and can't pay my rent? I'll be out on the street and never be able to get back on my feet again. I'd be too embarrassed to ask my family and friends for help. I'd be at the mercy of strangers.*

Identify the distorted thoughts. The distorted thoughts are *A faltering economy will result in the loss of my job* and *Losing my job would leave me destitute and helpless.*

Question their validity. *How likely am I really to lose my job? Suppose I did. Would I really wind up homeless? Would I really have no way of picking myself up? Would it really be impossible to ask for help from family and friends?*

Replace them with more realistic ones. *My company is showing no signs of real financial distress, and even if I did lose my job, I'd have ways of coping. Most people are still working, and I could find another job. I'm hardworking and good at what I do. I have supportive family members and friends whom I've helped in the past. If I couldn't pay my rent, I could stay with them until I got back on my feet. I have a little savings and, if worst came to worst, I could cash in my 401(k) plan. Also, I could receive unemployment for a while if I were laid off. It would be difficult, but not insurmountable.*

Challenging Unrealistic Fears

The above three examples illustrate how fear-producing cata-strophic thoughts can be challenged and countered by more real-istic, less anxious thinking. Now it's your turn. To challenge your unrealistic fears and replace them with more realistic thoughts is a five-part process:

1. Recognize your fearful thoughts. They usually begin with *What if. . . .*

2. Turn those thoughts into affirmative statements.

3. Subject those statements to a reality check—ques-tion their validity.

4. Formulate more realistic thoughts.

5. Put together a list of coping options that you would have if the feared event came to pass.

Exercise: Challenging Unrealistic Fears

On a blank piece of paper, write:

What I was telling myself (what-ifs)

Distorted thoughts

Challenge my distortions

More realistic thoughts

If the worst did happen, what could I do to cope?

Leave yourself room to write after each item. Before writ-ing, make at least twenty copies of the worksheet, since you will use it many times. Once you've made copies of the worksheet, follow the steps below to counter unrealistic thoughts associated with any fearful situation or worry.

Step 1: What I was telling myself

Pick a time when you're relatively relaxed and calm. If you're feeling anxious or upset, do something to relax, such as abdominal breathing or progressive muscle relaxation (see chapter 1). It's easier to notice your internal dialogue when you take time to slow down and relax.

After you get somewhat relaxed, ask yourself, *What was I telling myself that made me anxious?* Remember that these thoughts often start with *What if.* For example, if you fear driving on a freeway, your thought might be *What if I panic and lose control of the car?* Write your what-if statements under the first subhead of the worksheet: *What I was telling myself.*

Step 2: Distorted thoughts (change what-if statements to regular affirmative statements)

To make your distorted thoughts more clear and easy to challenge, change them from what-if statements to affirmative statements. For example, *What if I panic and lose control of the car?* would become *I'll panic and lose control of the car.* Write your revised thoughts under the second subhead of the worksheet: *Distorted patterns of thought.*

Step 3: Challenge my distortions

Remember that anxiety-producing fears and phobias are fueled by an overestimation of the probability of the feared outcome and an underestimation of your ability to cope if that outcome became reality. Challenge the distortions in your thoughts by asking questions such as:

- *What are the realistic odds of this happening?*

- *How often has this happened in the past?*

- *Am I viewing this situation as completely unmanageable or unsurvivable?*

When you do this, you subject your fears to a reality test and are better able to identify the distortions that they rest on. Write your answers to these questions under the subhead *Challenge my distortions.* For example, *It is not likely that I'll lose control of the car if I panic.*

Step 4: Formulate a more realistic thought

Use your answers to the questions in step 3 to formulate a more realistic thought. This thought should contain language and logic that reflects more balanced, realistic thinking. Write this thought under the subhead *More realistic thoughts*. For example, *If I started to feel panic while I was on the freeway, I'd definitely have ways to cope. My symptoms would be uncomfortable, but they would not make me 'lose it.'*

Step 5: If the worst did happen, what could I do to cope?

Finally, think about ways you could cope if your worst fear happened. Write your ways of coping under the subhead *If the worst did happen, what could I do to cope?* For example, *The moment I felt my anxiety getting severe, I could pull over to the shoulder on the side of the road and stop. If there wasn't a shoulder, I could slow down in the right lane, perhaps to forty-five miles per hour, put my flashers on, use coping statements and abdominal breathing to reduce my anxiety, and then get off at the nearest exit.*

Reread the realistic thoughts and ways you could cope with the worst-case scenario many times over a few weeks. This will reinforce them strongly in your mind. You might want to rewrite these statements on an index card that you keep with you and can pull out at a moment's notice. Repeat all of the steps of this exercise, using a separate copy of the worksheet, for each of your fears, phobias, or worries.

Quick Techniques for Coping

Changing the irrational beliefs that underlie and perpetuate panic, worry, and phobias is a key skill in anxiety control. It takes time and practice to master this skill, but once you do, you have a powerful tool at your fingertips.

There are other coping techniques that aren't as critical but can be helpful if used the minute you feel anxiety creeping up.

The lists below offer bite-size techniques that you can use to neutralize the early symptoms of anxiety. They can be used by themselves or as a precursor to the exercises in this chapter.

QUICK TECHNIQUES FOR COPING WITH PANIC

The techniques below are designed to cut short panic while it is still in its early stages. Try using them when you are in the Initial Stimulus or Worry Thoughts stages of the panic cycle (see the *Panic Sequence* section earlier in this chapter). If they don't provide relief at first, keep practicing them until you increase your proficiency.

- Engage in abdominal breathing for three to five minutes.

- Talk to a supportive person nearby or by phone.

- Get up and move around. Walk outdoors. Engage in your favorite type of exercise. Do household chores.

- Repeat your favorite coping statement for a minute or two. Try combining repetition of a coping statement with abdominal breathing. If you get bored with a particular statement, switch to another. (Alternatively, read down a prepared list of coping statements.)

- Stay in the present moment. Allow yourself to accept—not resist—what's happening. Abdominal breathing and focusing on your body (particularly your arms and legs) may help.

- Get angry at your anxiety. Shout at it with statements like *Get out of my way—I have things to do!* or *You're not going to run my life!* Pound a pillow with both fists if necessary.

- Experience something immediately pleasurable. Have a significant other or friend hold you. Take a hot shower. Sing a favorite song.

QUICK TECHNIQUES FOR COPING WITH WORRY

When you worry about something, it's easy to get caught in a spiral of frightening thoughts that increase your anxiety. The following techniques will help you divert your attention and energy away from your worry thoughts. They work best with low levels of anxiety or obsessive worry. Again, the more your practice them, the better you'll be at maximizing their potential usefulness.

- Do physical exercise, outdoors if possible.

- Do progressive muscle relaxation (see chapter 1).

- Talk to someone about something other than the worry, unless you want to express your feelings about it.

- Use visual distractions like TV, videos, your computer, or board games.

- Do something physical with your hands, like arts and crafts, repairing something, or gardening.

- Divert your obsessiveness to a jigsaw puzzle, crossword, or any type of puzzle you prefer.

- Take action on the issue that causes you worry. If you're afraid of flying, read a book or listen to a tape on overcoming that fear. If you're afraid of public speaking, practice giving your talk to a tape recorder.

TECHNIQUES FOR CHANGING YOUR PERSPECTIVE

The techniques below are designed to help you change your perspective on a problem or worrisome situation. They are designed to help you reframe your perception of whatever it is that's bothering you and shift your outlook from a negative, worry-producing one to a more positive and reassuring one. Not all of these techniques will be equally useful to you. Experiment with them and choose the ones that are most effective. Attitude shifts sometimes happen quickly, but you may also find it helpful to take time to relax first before you reframe your perspective.

- Surrender to the fact that the situation is the way it is whether you like it or not.

- Acknowledge that it would be okay to lighten up about it.

- Expand your compassion for all people who experience similar things—you're not alone.

- Cultivate a sense of fascination with it. Notice that it's at least interesting or novel.

- Be open to the problem making a contribution to you somehow. There may be something it's teaching you.

- Turn everything over to God.

- Imagine that working with the problem might strengthen your character.

- Feel the tingle of aliveness within the pattern of energy you've got going around the problem. Focus on just the energy itself. After a while it may shift.

- Trust that you are strong enough to handle even the worst of this.

- Realize that it's very likely not as bad as your worst thoughts about it.

- Be very gentle, patient, and caring with yourself in the presence of your feelings.

- Consider whether some part of you might actually rather have the problem than change.

- Acknowledge that you've struggled with this about long enough and that trying to control it may not be your best strategy.

- Welcome this as an opportunity to let go of ego.

- See the problem possibly as a metaphor for your entire life.

- Trust that since other people have made it through this, you can too.

- Acknowledge that what's bothering you is not what really matters the most in life anyway.

- Notice that if you're doing your best, that's the best you can do anyway.

- Trust in the inevitability of this passing. Affirm *This too will pass.*

- Breathe more deeply and just be with it. Trust that in a while, it will shift.

 5

Physical Conditions That Can Aggravate Anxiety

It's likely that rather than having one identifiable cause, your anxiety springs from a mosaic of lifestyle, physical, and psychological factors. In this chapter we'll look at some common physical conditions that can aggravate anxiety or tax your system and make you more vulnerable to its effects. These conditions include *adrenal exhaustion, candidiasis, body toxicity, premenstrual syndrome,* and *seasonal affective disorder. Hypoglycemia* and *food allergies,* discussed in chapter 3, can have similar effects. While these conditions are not at all uncommon, it is often difficult to identify their symptoms. Anyone who suffers from anxiety should be aware of the symptoms, treatments, and causes of the disorders discussed in this chapter.

Adrenal Exhaustion

Prolonged and unremitting stress taxes your adrenal glands. Hans Selye, a well-known expert on stress, has described how protracted stress on the adrenal glands results in a state of chronic underfunctioning or exhaustion (1984). Insufficient adrenal resources, in turn, tend to affect how you handle stressful situations, making it more likely that you will become anxious in the face of stress. Inadequate sleep; life stresses of all kinds; prolonged exposure to heat or cold; exposure to toxins, pollutants, or substances you're allergic to; and taking cortisone over a period of time can also contribute to adrenal exhaustion. Sudden trauma or severe physical illness can initiate or worsen adrenal exhaustion. Notice that many of these factors, particularly sudden trauma such as losses or life transitions, also play a role in the onset of anxiety disorders. Anxiety disorders and adrenal exhaustion frequently occur together.

Adrenal exhaustion develops in stages. When you're combating stress, the adrenal glands tend to hyperfunction, producing large amounts of adrenaline and noradrenaline as well as steroid hormones such as *cortisol*. As stress becomes prolonged, the glands begin to be overtaxed and go into a state of temporary underfunctioning. If you are relatively healthy, the glands will try to compensate and can actually rebuild themselves to the point of *hypertrophy* (growing larger). However, if high levels of stress continue, the glands will eventually exhaust themselves again and then remain in a chronic state of underfunctioning. At this stage they can oscillate between overproducing adrenaline, which can cause panic or mood swings, and underproducing adrenaline, which is associated with fatigue and poor stress tolerance. The ultimate outcome of prolonged adrenal exhaustion can be health problems such as chronic fatigue syndrome, fibromyalgia, chronic bronchitis or sinusitis, and autoimmune disorders ranging from lupus to rheumatoid arthritis.

Symptoms of adrenal exhaustion include:

- low stress tolerance (little things that didn't use to bother you get to you)

- lethargy and fatigue (often manifested in difficulty getting up in the morning)

- light-headedness when standing up quickly (called *postural hypotension*)

- light sensitivity (difficulty adjusting to bright light outdoors)

- difficulties with concentration and memory

- insomnia

- hypoglycemia

- allergies (to foods, environmental substances, pollens, molds, etc.)

- increased symptoms of premenstrual syndrome

- more frequent colds and respiratory conditions

Hypoglycemia and adrenal exhaustion. Hypoglycemia and adrenal exhaustion often go hand in hand. The adrenals function along with the pancreas in helping to maintain stable blood sugar levels. When the adrenals underfunction, blood sugar levels tend to become erratic. As adrenal fatigue worsens, the immune system is compromised, leading to increased susceptibility to allergies, asthma, respiratory infections, and colds.

Addictions and adrenal exhaustion. Addiction to caffeine, tobacco, alcohol, or recreational drugs is frequently associated with adrenal exhaustion, as is the physiological craving for sugar. Continued use of any of these substances tends to worsen the condition. If you have any of these addictions, your risk of adrenal insufficiency is higher than average.

Your day-to-day life and adrenal exhaustion. A day-to-day life that is chronically stressful and demanding due to perfectionism and self-imposed pressure to achieve also often leads to adrenal exhaustion.

RECOVERY FROM ADRENAL EXHAUSTION

To recover from adrenal exhaustion, you have to address it on several different fronts. Certain lifestyle changes, supplementation, and dietary modifications can be helpful. These are outlined below.

Simplify your life. Ask yourself which of your habits, practices, and obligations clutter your life rather than enrich it (see chapter 9).

Regularly practice your preferred form of relaxation. Whether this is progressive muscle relaxation, guided visualization, yoga, or meditation, try to commit to practice it daily.

Give yourself downtime daily. Remember that downtime is not a luxury, it is necessary for maintaining a vibrant, fulfilling life (see chapter 1). Break up your day with two or three twenty- to thirty-minute periods of relaxation.

Strive to get eight hours of sleep at night. Sufficient sleep is not a luxury, either. Turn in by 10:00 or 11:00 P.M. if possible. Whenever you can sleep late in the morning, let yourself do so.

Exercise regularly. Get twenty to thirty minutes of moderate exercise every day, preferably outdoors (see chapter 2).

Eliminate caffeine, nicotine, alcohol, and recreational drugs. Substitute herb teas for caffeinated beverages. Licorice tea is especially good if you're hypoglycemic.

For three months, eliminate all forms of sugar. Use xylitol or stevia to sweeten foods or beverages. Eliminating sugar means cutting out white and brown sugar, honey, chocolate, molasses, corn syrup, maple syrup, and dried fruit. Substitute fresh fruits in moderation. Xylitol is a sweetner that is made from the fiber of the birch tree. It produces only a small increase in blood sugar and no rise in insulin levels. Stevia is derived from a South American herb and is many times sweeter than sugar. It has no calories and is much safer than artifical sweetners like aspartame and saccharin. After three months, you can reintroduce natural sugars such as honey in very small amounts.

Eat a healthy, balanced diet. As much as possible, eliminate processed foods and foods to which you're allergic. Emphasize whole grains, fresh vegetables, and fresh fruits in your diet. Eat protein in the form of beans and grains; eggs; organic poultry; free-range, hormone- and antibiotic-free meat; or fish. Do not overeat carbohydrates. Reduce your consumption of simple carbohydrates such as pasta, bread, chips, potatoes, cereal, crackers, rolls, etc. Combine a fat, protein, and complex carbohydrate source at every meal. Avoid eating just fruit first thing in the morning and avoid fruit juices (see chapter 3).

If you have hypoglycemia, eat the appropriate diet. Be sure to eat a protein-carbohydrate snack two to three hours after each main meal (see chapter 3).

SUPPLEMENTS FOR ADRENAL EXHAUSTION

Certain supplements can help relieve adrenal exhaustion. Talk to your health professional about taking the supplements and quantities listed below:

- Vitamin C with bioflavonoids: 500 to 1,000 milligrams three times per day with meals

- Zinc: 30 milligrams daily

- Chromium picolinate: 200 to 400 milligrams daily

- Vitamin B_6 in the form of P5P (pyridoxyl-5-phosphate): 50 milligrams twice daily

- Calcium with magnesium (preferably in chelated forms such as citrate or aspartate): 1,000 milligrams calcium and 500 to 1,000 milligrams magnesium at bedtime

- Pantothenic acid: 500 milligrams once or twice daily

- Adrenal cortex glandulars: Consult your physician, naturopath, or health practitioner. These supplements can be helpful in treating adrenal exhaustion and are preferable to taking *whole* adrenal glandular supplements.

Candidiasis

Candidiasis or "yeast syndrome" is the result of an overgrowth of a particular yeast, *Candida albicans,* in the intestinal tract, genitourinary tract, or both. Normally, candida lives in a healthy balance with bacteria in the gut, but certain conditions can lead it to multiply, first proliferating throughout the intestinal tract and then moving beyond the gut to invade tissues and organ systems throughout the body. Candidiasis affects a lot of people, especially women.

In the early stages of candidiasis, localized infections—particularly skin rashes and "yeast infections" (vaginitis)—are common. Other symptoms include:

- chronic fungal infections such as athlete's foot, ringworm, or jock itch

- fatigue or feeling drained

- depression or mood swings

- gastrointestinal problems such as bloating, cramps, chronic diarrhea, or constipation

- chronic anxiety and tension

- food allergies

- poor memory

- headaches

- rectal itching

- extreme sensitivity to chemicals, perfumes, or tobacco smoke

- severe premenstrual syndrome symptoms

- muscle or joint pain

- cravings for sweets, bread, or alcohol

A characteristic feature of candidiasis is that the symptoms worsen after you eat sugar or drink alcohol. All forms of sugar (except for xylitol) and alcohol feed the yeast and cause it to spread. Symptoms also tend to worsen in damp, moldy climates or environments. If you have five or more of the above symptoms, you may be dealing with candidiasis. If you have two or three of these symptoms, you may want to consult with a health professional to rule out the possibility of this problem.

WHAT CAUSES CANDIDIASIS?

Factors that increase your risk of developing candidiasis include frequent use of broad-spectrum antibiotics such as ampicillin, amoxicillin, Ceclor (cefaclon), Bactrim (sulfamethoxazole), or Septra (sulfamethoxazole and trimethoprim) in the past; having used birth control pills for more than a year; frequent or prolonged use of steroid hormones such as cortisone, prednisone, or other corticosteroids; living in a damp, moldy environment; heavy consumption of sweets or alcohol; and having certain diseases such as diabetes, cancer, or AIDS.

DIAGNOSING CANDIDIASIS

There are three ways of diagnosing candidiasis. One is to use a diagnostic questionnaire such as the one developed by Kenneth Crook in his classic book, *The Yeast Connection*. Alternatively, your doctor can measure antibodies to candida (IgG, IgM, and IgA) with a blood test. Elevated IgG antibody levels indicate that the candida organism has proliferated to excessively high levels in the gut. Elevated IgM antibodies indicate that the candida has ventured beyond the intestine and become systemic. High levels of IgA antibodies are indicative of mucosal involvement, such as in vaginal yeast infections. Candidiasis can also be diagnosed through a stool analysis, which may show high levels of the yeast. However, the stool test may be negative even when other indications are present.

RECOVERY FROM CANDIDIASIS

Recovery from chronic candidiasis can be achieved with a three-pronged program. First, for three months, eliminate from your diet foods that the candida organism feeds on. This includes all kinds of sugar except xylitol or stevia: sucrose, fructose, dextrose, maltose, galactose, dried fruits, and fruit juices. (Xylitol and stevia do not feed candida.) Alcohol, yeast, fermented foods, cheese, vinegar, and refined flour products (including bread) should also be avoided, as they feed candida too. After three months you can reintroduce these foods in small quantities. See the *Candida Diet* section below.

Second, it is often necessary to take an antifungal medication such as nystatin or Nizoral (ketoconazole), which would be prescribed by your doctor, for a period of several months. Note that there is some controversy among health practitioners about the use of these drugs. Medical doctors are often more inclined to use these drugs in high doses, whereas some naturopaths and alternative health practitioners use nystatin modestly or not at all. One problem is that nystatin kills candida only in the gut and does not directly affect systemic proliferation. Another is that after you use nystatin long-term, the yeast may mutate to other forms which are resistant to the drug. An alternative to nystatin used by some health practitioners is *caprylic acid.* Since it is absorbed through the intestine, it can have a greater effect on systemic candidiasis. In addition, many practitioners use goldenseal and/or grapefruit seed extract. These plants contain *berberine,* which battles candida. Some people also like to add pau d'arco tea to their treatment program because of its antibacterial and fungicidal properties. Taking a multivitamin and multimineral capsule, vitamin C, Vitamin E, and zinc can also be helpful, as can increasing your intake of essential fatty acids. Discuss these options with your doctor, and remember that they should be used in conjunction with the candida diet.

Finally, candida tends to crowd out healthy intestinal bacteria, so you need to restore normal bacterial ecology in the intestine by implanting useful bacteria such as *Lactobacillus acidophilus* and *Lactobacillus bifidus*. Probiotic supplements are usually part of the treatment. Talk to your doctor about these. After one to three months on this regimen, you should be retested to see if your candida levels have returned to normal.

The Candida Diet

The following are dietary principles to help in the recovery from candidiasis. You may need to modify them to fit your particular needs or lifestyle, but in general they provide a good rule of thumb.

Foods that should be *avoided* include:

- milk and other dairy products

- sweets and all forms of sugar, except xylitol or stevia

- alcohol

- fruit and fruit juices (with the possible exception of grapefruit)

- honey, molasses, artificial sweeteners

- chocolate

- foods containing yeast, including all forms of bread made with yeast

- aged cheese

- peanut butter

- smoked or processed nuts

- vinegar

- mushrooms

- carrot juice

- peanuts

- starchy foods, such as pastas, chips, or potatoes, in large quantities

- leftovers (except if they've been frozen)

The following are foods that you should *include* in your diet:

- chicken or fish

- raw or cooked vegetables

- grains in moderation (whole-grain rice is preferable to wheat)

- eggs

- beans

- lemon- or oil-based salad dressings (without vinegar)

- raw nuts

- yeast-free breads (available in most health food stores)

- unaged cheeses (such as Monterey Jack)

- garlic

- enteric-coated volatile oil preparations (for example, oregano oil)

Some people call the candida diet the "can't eat it" diet because it seems so restrictive. If you're used to eating large quantities of sweets, you may find yourself calling it this in the week or so after you begin. After a few weeks, however, you'll find that a diet free of sugar can still be enjoyable, and your cravings will begin to dissipate.

If you are like many people who successfully recover from candidiasis, you will find that you have increased energy, less depression, fewer gastrointestinal problems, and more overall vitality. These benefits will make the dietary trade-offs easier to bear.

Body Toxicity

Excessive body toxicity may not directly increase anxiety, but it adds to the physical stress level of your body and thus makes the impact of anxiety symptoms greater. Body toxicity often aggravates allergies and chemical sensitivities, which in turn can aggravate anxiety. Factors that can cause toxins to build up in your body include consumption of chemicals, additives, and pesticides in food; exposure to environmental pollutants in the air and water; exposure to substances used indoors, such as household cleaners, deodorants, hairsprays, cosmetics, and even carpeting (which may outgas toxic chemicals); use of either prescription or recreational drugs; and buildup of your own metabolic waste products, which are produced in abundance when you're under stress.

If you have reached a high level of cumulative toxicity you may experience any of the following symptoms frequently:

- fatigue and low energy

- joint or muscle pain

- headaches

- "brain fog" or mental confusion

- irritability and moodiness

- insomnia

- sensitivity to chemicals in the environment

- depression or irritability

- heavily coated tongue or abnormal body odor

- excess mucus (coughing and wheezing)

- allergies

- sinus or respiratory problems

The liver and colon are the organs most affected by toxic buildup. Next to the brain and heart, the liver is probably the most important organ in your body. It is the metabolic "factory" in which hundreds of functions necessary for life take place. Some of the more important ones include:

- filtration of the blood

- secretion of bile, which is necessary to digest fats

- extraction and storage of vitamins (such as vitamins A, D, and E) from nutrients in your bloodstream

- synthesis of fatty acids from amino acids and sugar

- oxidation of fat to produce energy

- storage of sugar in the form of *glycogen,* which can be used when the body is depleted of blood sugar or glucose

- detoxification of the by-products of digestion (such as ammonia from protein digestion)

- detoxification of metabolic waste products as well as all chemicals and foreign substances to which you are exposed

Exposure to toxins, some drugs, poor diet, and overeating can cause accumulations of fatty deposits in the liver and interfere with its functioning. Regular consumption of large quantities of alcohol can damage the liver and eventually lead to cirrhosis. Chronic overeating forces the liver to work harder and may weaken it over time, especially if you are eating foods laden with preservatives and additives. Eating a lot of fried or processed foods containing trans fats can also be hard on the liver.

DETOXIFYING YOUR LIFESTYLE

There are several dietary and lifestyle changes you can make to decrease the level of toxicity in your body.

Avoid foods containing preservatives and additives. Try to eat unprocessed, whole foods as much as possible. Be sure to include plenty of fresh fruits and vegetables, preferably five servings a day.

Reduce or eliminate caffeine, nicotine, sugar, and alcohol. Aside from other health problems these substances can cause, they leave toxic waste products in your body.

Minimize your use of drugs. Take only necessary medications prescribed by your physician and avoid recreational drug use.

Reduce animal proteins (especially red meat) and increase vegetable sources of protein (tofu, tempeh, and beans). When metabolized, animal proteins can produce toxic by-products, especially if not properly digested.

Drink purified or filtered water. Eight eight-ounce glasses a day will assist your kidneys in their natural process of elimination. Your kidneys are critically involved in ridding your body of various toxic waste products.

Include ample fiber in your diet. Make sure your diet contains high-fiber foods such as whole-grain cereals, all kinds of bran, most fresh fruits, fresh raw vegetables, nuts and seeds, and legumes such as beans, lentils, or peas. You may also want to take a fiber supplement recommended by your health practitioner.

Move away from acid-forming, congestive foods toward more alkaline-forming, detoxifying foods. This means reducing your consumption of red meat, sweets, fried foods, fatty foods, milk, cheese, eggs, refined flour, salty foods, as well as any foods you know you're allergic to such as wheat or dairy.

Increase your consumption of fresh vegetables, fruits, whole grains, beans, nuts, and seeds, and increase the proportion of raw to cooked foods that you eat. It's good to have some raw, fresh vegetables or fruit at each meal. Be aware that the degree to which you move from acid- to alkaline-forming foods should be tailored to your individual constitution and needs. If you've been highly toxic in your eating habits, make the change gradually. Have one day a week in which you lighten your diet.

Get regular, vigorous exercise. This helps to clear your body of toxins through sweating, and it aids the digestive, renal, and lymphatic systems.

Discuss the use of antioxidant supplements with your doctor or health practitioner. These supplements include vitamin C, vitamin E, beta-carotene, selenium, zinc, lipoic acid, coenzyme Q_{10}, and amino acids such as cysteine, methionine, glututhione, and glycine.

Investigate various herbs that can help detoxify your body. Consult a naturally oriented physician or herbologist before using herbs for detoxicification. Some herbs believed to aid detoxification are milk thistle, dandelion root, burdock, cayenne, ginger, licorice, echinacea, and goldenseal. A high-potency multivitamin and mineral supplement can help combat heavy metal poisoning and help the liver detoxify.

Support colon detoxification. Consider a natural laxative, which may contain bentonite, senna, or cascara sagrada. Psyllium seed husks, available in most health food stores, also cleanse mucus along the small intestine and pull toxins from both the small and large intestines. Discuss these options with your doctor or health practitioner. Remember that even natural laxatives can be habit-forming, so use them sparingly. Some people report benefits from receiving *colonics* from a certified colon therapist. In a colonic, your colon is irrigated and cleansed with water using a special machine.

Support liver detoxification. Eat foods that protect the liver and improve its function. These include vegetables in the *brassica* family, such as cabbage, broccoli, and brussels sprouts, and high-sulfur foods like garlic, onions, eggs, and legumes. Herbs such as dandelion root, burdock, and milk thistle are often used to help detoxify the liver.

HEAVY METAL TOXICITY

Metals such as mercury, lead, and aluminum have no safe amount in the human body. Unfortunately, as a result of modern industrial pollution and other sources, people are exposed to heavy metals in excessive amounts. This can generate a wide variety of symptoms. The severity of the problem is dependent on the type of metal, your age, the extent of your exposure, and the presence of protective factors that inhibit absorption and mitigate the long-range effects of the metal. A simple hair analysis test, which can be performed by your doctor or health practitioner, will give you a clear indication of whether you have a problem. In a hair analysis test, a small sample of your hair is sent to a lab, which analyzes it both for excesses of heavy metals such as mercury, lead, cadmium, nickel, and aluminum as well as for deficiencies of essential minerals such as calcium, magnesium, zinc, and manganese.

Mercury Toxicity

Mercury is the most toxic of all heavy metals. It is a cumulative poison, retained not only in the body but in the brain. The two most common sources of excess mercury are dental amalgams and certain types of fish.

Most so-called silver dental fillings are in fact up to 50 percent mercury. As the fillings age, they may release mercury vapor, which combines with chemicals in the mouth to create small amounts of the toxic compound *methyl mercury*. This in turn is absorbed directly into your body.

Nearly all fish contain trace amounts of methyl mercury, but large predator fish such as sharks, swordfish, marlins, and larger tuna tend to accumulate higher levels as a result of eating copious amounts of smaller fish. If you eat large sea or freshwater fish frequently (more than two or three times per week), you may be at risk for elevated mercury levels. Other sources of mercury exposure include fabric softeners, inks used by printers or from tattoos, some paints, polishes, solvents, and wood preservatives.

Symptoms of mercury toxicity include fatigue, irritability, insomnia, memory loss, confusion, anxiety, depression, muscular weakness, and decreased immunity. In more severe cases, numbness, tingling, and symptoms which mimic multiple sclerosis may appear.

Lead Toxicity

Lead is one of the most widely used metals in the modern world and also one of the most toxic. Like mercury, it tends to accumulate in the body and is not easily excreted. It inhibits a variety of enzyme functions, and, when present in toxic amounts, can damage the kidneys, liver, heart, and nervous system. Children absorb 20 to 45 percent more lead per pound of body weight than do adults, and so are particularly vulnerable. If you are deficient in calcium, you are also more susceptible to lead toxicity.

Sources of lead exposure include lead-based paints, ceramic glazes, leaded gasoline, lead-acid batteries in cars, tobacco, some imported and domestic wines, and fruits and vegetables in lead-soldered cans. Water supplied through lead pipes can also be a problem (lead piping was used in most homes before 1930). More recent copper pipes are often assembled with lead solder, which is 50 percent lead. So in general, it's a good idea to have a water purification system that filters out lead. Lead poisoning is unfortunately common in children in inner cities, who are exposed to toxic fumes in higher quantities and may also eat chips of lead-based paints which have peeled off walls. Around 200 children in the United States die each year from lead poisoning, and about 800 suffer permanent brain damage.

General symptoms of lead toxicity include fatigue, irritability, anxiety, mental confusion, loss of appetite, weight loss, tremors, seizures, and dizziness. Symptoms of lead toxicity in children include poor bone growth, learning disabilities, muscle weakness, and bouts of gastrointestinal colic.

Aluminum Toxicity

Aluminum is not a heavy metal, but it can be toxic to the body in excessive amounts, especially if it is deposited in the brain. The symptoms of aluminum toxicity mimic those of Alzheimer's disease. In addition to affecting the brain, excess aluminum can damage your kidneys.

The overuse of antacids containing aluminum hydroxide is the most common cause of aluminum toxicity in the modern world. It's highly recommended that you use antacids that do not contain aluminum hydroxide. Other sources of aluminum exposure include aluminum cookware, many everyday household products (such as antiperspirants and baking powder) that contain aluminum, and municipal water supplies that are treated with alum (aluminum sulfate).

Symptoms of aluminum toxicity include extreme nervousness, headaches, forgetfulness and memory loss, muscle weakness, gastrointestinal disturbances, anemia, decreased liver and kidney function, and softening of the bones.

TREATMENT FOR MERCURY, LEAD, AND ALUMINUM TOXICITY

If mercury levels are only mildly elevated, nutrients such as lipoic acid, n-acetyl cysteine, and phosphatidylcholine may be helpful. Otherwise, the primary treatment for both mercury and lead toxicity is *chelation therapy,* most commonly using *DMSA* (meso-2,3-dimercaptosuccinic acid). DMSA binds with mercury and lead, which are then excreted from the body through urine and feces. It is usually taken in oral form (capsules). Chelation should be done only under the supervision of a physician or experienced health practitioner. Treatment usually consists of taking 200 to 1,200 milligrams of DMSA for two or three days, followed by a two-week wash-out period, and then repeating the treatment as many times as necessary until mercury or lead levels come down to within normal range.

For mercury toxicity, supplements such as the amino acids n-acteyl cysteine and methionine, chlorella (a green algae that has been demonstrated to remove heavy metals from the body), and fresh cilantro may be recommended along with a whole-foods diet and large quantities of filtered water. For lead toxicity, additional supplements such as apple pectin, alfalfa, kelp, or garlic may be recommended. The chelation process may take one to three months. Hair analyses are subsequently given to retest mercury or lead levels.

Chelation therapy is also used to treat aluminum toxicity. However, some doctors believe that it is ineffective for aluminum and recommend other methods of removing aluminum from the body. Check with your doctor or health practitioner on current detoxification procedures.

Most doctors recommend that you have your "silver" dental fillings replaced with composite fillings before the chelation procedure. If the mercury fillings are your primary source of mercury exposure, it makes sense to have them removed before proceeding with mercury detoxification. In most major metropolitan areas, there are dentists who specialize in the delicate process of removing and replacing mercury dental amalgams in such a way as to minimize further mercury exposure. Consult with a holistic physician or naturopath in your area to get a referral to such a dentist.

Premenstrual Syndrome

Premenstrual syndrome (PMS) involves a constellation of disruptive physical and psychological symptoms that many women experience in the days or week prior to menstruation. Common physical symptoms include water retention, breast soreness, bloating, acne, headaches, increased hunger, and craving for sweets. Psychological symptoms can include depression, irritability, anxiety and tension, mood swings, distractibility and forgetfulness, fatigue, and even a feeling of "going crazy." Up to half of all women experience a premenstrual increase in depression, anxiety, or irritability in addition to some of the above physical symptoms. Panic reactions can also be a symptom of PMS. The question to ask is whether your panic attacks typically occur—or increase in frequency and intensity—during the days before menstruation. If so, treating your PMS may help to reduce or eliminate panic attacks.

Most medical theories about PMS relate to an imbalance in the amount of estrogen and progesterone in a woman's body, particularly during the second half of the menstrual cycle. During this fourteen-day period, progesterone levels normally fall, while estrogen levels may rise slightly. Insufficient levels of progesterone relative to the amount of estrogen tend to promote water retention and other problematic symptoms of PMS.

Other theories about PMS suggest that menstruation allows the body to throw off excess toxins accumulated through improper diet as well as from exposure to environmental contaminants and pollutants. Thus the symptoms experienced just prior to menstruation reflect the body's reaction to excess toxicity. The implication is that eating a healthy diet and reducing exposure to other toxins should help lessen PMS symptoms.

Both theories are probably valid. PMS symptoms can definitely be helped by eliminating foods that tend to aggravate them. Symptoms can also be alleviated in many cases with the aid of supplemental vitamins, minerals, and herbs, particularly those that raise the body's level of progesterone. Recommendations for treating PMS follow. Before undertaking any of them, consult a physician, nutritionist, or qualified practitioner of Chinese medicine who is well versed in treating this problem.

DIETARY HELP FOR PMS

Avoid or minimize the following foods:

- Foods high in sugar as well as large amounts of simple carbohydrates (bread, chips, or pasta). It's especially important to avoid the impulse to binge on sweets and carbohydrate foods, including chocolate, for one week before the expected onset of symptoms.

- Salty foods. This will help reduce bloating and water retention.

- High-fat foods.

- Caffeinated drinks, including coffee, tea, and colas. Caffeine is linked to breast tenderness.

- Alcohol.

Eat plenty of fresh fruits and vegetables, whole-grain breads and cereals, and legumes, nuts, free-range poultry, and fish.

SUPPLEMENTS FOR PMS

What follows is a list of vitamin and mineral supplements that can help relieve PMS symptoms.

A high-potency B-complex in conjunction with calcium and magnesium (1,000 milligrams calcium to 500 milligrams magnesium). Supplementing with calcium and magnesium may help reduce menstrual cramps.

Vitamin B$_6$. The recommended dose is 200 milligrams daily during the week before menstruation, but you should avoid taking this much vitamin B$_6$ for more than one week out of every month.

Essential fatty acids. A good source of essential fatty acids can be found in fish oils, which contain both *EPA* and *DHA* omega-3 fatty acids. You can take 500 to 2000 milligrams per day of combined EPA/DHA in the form of fish oil capsules. An alternative is flax oil or flaxmeal, which provides a plant-based form of omega-3 fatty acids. However, the conversion to EPA and DHA is nowhere near as efficient as occurs with the fish oils. Borage oil, black currant seed oil, or evening primrose oil are sources of

GLA, a special omega-6 fatty acid that is essential for humans. You can take 300-900 milligrams of any one of these daily.

Natural progesterone: Available in skin creams that can be bought over the counter. A common dose is 1 ounce per month, the equivalent of one quarter teaspoon daily, skipping the first seven days of your cycle. We recommend consulting with a health practitioner skilled in treating PMS when you first start to use natural progesterone.

Tryptophan in the form of 5-HTP or L-Tryptophan (see chapter 6), taken at least on the days you expereince symptoms. PMS is often associated with reduced serotonin activity, and tryptophan will boost your serotonin levels.

HERBS FOR PMS

The following herbs can help reduce the physical and psychological symptoms of PMS:

- Dong quai *(Angelica sinensis)*. This herb can boost energy and stabilize your mood during PMS. It can be taken in capsule form (follow dosage recommendations given on the label) or as a tea.

- Ginger root or licorice root.

- Rosemary, cramp bark, and kava have been known to reduce cramps. (See the caveat about Kava in chapter 6.)

- Kombucha tea. This provides energy and stimulates the immune system. It has been reported to be helpful for some women.

REGULAR EXERCISE

Last but not least, a program of regular physical exercise will liven up your metabolism and reduce stress levels. If you can't do vigorous exercise, try walking at least one mile each day. See chapter 2.

Seasonal Affective Disorder

When the seasons change from spring and summer to fall and winter, do you develop the following symptoms?

- lower energy than usual

- awakening feeling tired, although you sleep more

- mood changes such as feeling more anxious, irritable, sad, or depressed

- diminished productivity or creativity

- feeling that you have little control over your appetite or weight

- more memory and concentration problems

- lowered interest in socializing

- lessened ability to cope with stress

- less enthusiasm about the future or reduced enjoyment in your life

If you said yes to two or more of these, you may be one of the many people affected by *seasonal affective disorder* (SAD) or a milder form of this disorder known as *subsyndromal* SAD. Seasonal affective disorder is a cyclical depression that occurs during the winter months, typically between November and March. It's brought on by insufficient exposure to light. As the days get shorter and the angle of the sun changes during fall, the symptoms of SAD begin to appear. An estimated 20 percent of the American adult population, or 36 million people, are affected by SAD and subsyndromal SAD. The further from the equator you happen to live, the more susceptible you are.

ANXIETY AND SAD

Many individuals dealing with anxiety disorders experience an aggravation of their condition during the late fall and winter. Panic attacks may occur more often, and generalized anxiety may increase along with depression. It's not surprising that this is so, because the same systems of the brain that contribute to the neurobiological basis of depression, the *noradrenergic system* and the *serotonin system,* are also implicated in anxiety disorders, particularly panic disorder, generalized anxiety disorder, and obsessive-compulsive disorder. Biochemical imbalances in these systems tipped one way may cause depression; tipped the other way, they may aggravate anxiety disorders. And for many individuals, unfortunately, problems with anxiety and depression coexist, both becoming aggravated during the winter months.

Whether they manifest as depression or anxiety, the symptoms of SAD are caused by decreased availability of light. SAD can be aggravated not only by reduced light outside during the winter months but by spending too much time in indoor environments which have low levels of light, whether at home or work. SAD symptoms have been reported even in the summer among people who work in environments without windows. They can also occur in sensitive individuals at any time of year after a succession of cloudy days.

It used to be thought that SAD was caused by insufficient suppression of a hormone in the brain called *melatonin.* Melatonin is secreted by the pineal gland in the brain at night after several hours of darkness. It is one of the mechanisms by which your brain lets you know it is time to go to sleep. With light in the morning, melatonin secretion is suppressed, and you know that it's time to wake up. Although popular for many years, the hypothesis that SAD is caused by insufficient melatonin suppression has not been borne out by systematic research. Results of studies have been mixed, and researchers have looked in other directions to find clues to the cause of SAD. The hypothesis that is currently receiving the most attention is that light insufficiency can cause a reduction in levels of serotonin in the brain. Norman Rosenthal (1993), one of the leading researchers in this field, writes that when susceptible individuals are exposed to too little environmental light—such as during winter—they produce too little serotonin. Rosenthal and others believe that these low levels of serotonin are responsible for the symptoms of SAD.

Serotonin deficiencies are frequently associated with symptoms of depression, anxiety, or both; that is why drugs that block the reuptake of serotonin in the brain—drugs such as Prozac (fluoxetine), Zoloft (sertraline), or Paxil (paroxetine)—often alleviate depression and many of the anxiety disorders. But why should reduced light affect serotonin? And why only in certain individuals? The answer to the first question is still being researched. In answer to the second question, there is some evidence that people who are susceptible to SAD may be less able to receive or process light at a neurological level relative to people who do not develop SAD.

During the winter, people with SAD tend to crave sweets and carbohydrates. Eating large amounts of carbohydrates usually increases the amount of *tryptophan* (an essential amino acid derived naturally from protein foods) that gets into the brain. Once in the brain, tryptophan becomes serotonin, the neurotransmitter that is so critical to psychological well-being. Eating sweets and carbohydrates gives tryptophan a competitive edge over the body's other amino acids in getting into the brain. So, if you tend to be drawn to sweets and starches in the wintertime, it may be your body's attempt to raise your levels of serotonin.

LIGHT THERAPY FOR SAD

The treatment that most effectively reduces the symptoms of SAD is *light therapy*. In principle it would be possible to reduce SAD in the winter by spending prolonged periods of time outdoors every day. Unless you're a ski instructor or a snowplow operator, however, this is pretty impractical. Light therapy involves the use of one or more specific devices indoors to increase your exposure to bright light. Sometimes light-sensitive individuals can experience an improvement simply by increasing normal room light or installing brighter lightbulbs. However, most SAD sufferers seem to require exposure to higher light levels—at least four times brighter than normal household and office light.

Light boxes are commonly used to alleviate symptoms of SAD. A light box is a set of fluorescent bulbs in a box, with a diffusing plastic screen. Most of these devices deliver between 2,500 and 10,000 lux of light energy—considerably above the usual range of indoor lighting (approximately 200 to 1,000 lux). A typical light therapy session involves sitting within two or three feet of a light box for a period of half an hour to two hours in the morning. It's neither necessary nor advisable to look directly at the light; rather, you can use the time to read, write, eat, sew, or do whatever you need to do. The amount of daily light exposure needed to achieve a reduction in symptoms varies from one person to another. Experiment with varying the duration of exposure according to your own needs.

Other devices used in light therapy are *dawn simulators* and *light visors*. The dawn simulator creates an artificial dawn in your bedroom by having a light come on very dimly at, say, 6:00 A.M. and gradually brightening until 7:00 A.M. The light visor is a lightweight source of light which you can wear on your head. It allows you to have more mobility than the light box.

Light therapy is very effective when administered properly. In experimental trials, it has been shown to help 75 to 80 percent of SAD sufferers within a week if used regularly (Rosenthal 1993). Before undertaking light therapy on your own, you should consult with a physician or another health professional who is knowledgeable about this therapy and its application. Although light therapy devices are available without a prescription, you can save yourself time—as well as such possible side effects as headache, eyestrain, irritability, or insomnia—by getting assistance in using them properly. See the Resources appendix for more information about SAD and light therapy devices.

COPING WITH SAD

The National Organization for Seasonal Affective Disorder (NOSAD) offers the following suggestions:

- Discuss your symptoms with your physician. You may be referred to a psychiatrist who may diagnose seasonal affective disorder or subsyndromal SAD and prescribe special light treatments to help relieve your symptoms. Serotonin-boosting supplements such as tryptophan or Saint-John's-wort (see chapter 6) can be helpful in treating some people with seasonal depression.

- If you have a medical diagnosis of SAD or subsyndromal SAD and your doctor prescribes light treatment, do not skip or shorten treatment because you're feeling better; you may relapse. Work with your doctor in adjusting the length of time, time of day, distance, and intensity of light for your own individualized treatment.

- Get as much light as possible and avoid dark environments during daylight hours in winter.

- Reduce mild winter depressive symptoms by exercising daily, preferably outdoors, to take advantage of natural light.

- If you are unable to exercise outdoors in the winter due to extreme cold, exercise inside. If possible, try sitting in sunlight from a south-facing window for short but frequent periods during the day.

- Rearrange work spaces at home, and work near a window, or set up bright lights in your work area.

- Stay on a regular sleep-wake schedule. People with SAD report being more alert and less fatigued when they get up and go to sleep at preset hours than when they vary their schedules.

- Be aware of cold outside temperatures and dress to conserve energy and warmth. Many affected by seasonal changes report sensitivity to extreme temperatures.

- Arrange family outings and social occasions for daytime and early evening in winter. Avoid staying up late, which disrupts your sleep schedule and biological clock.

- Conserve energy by managing time wisely and avoiding or minimizing unnecessary stress.

- Try putting lights on a timer in your bedroom or use a dawn simulator set to switch on a half hour or more before you get up. Some people with SAD report that this light technique has an antidepressant effect and helps them awaken more easily.

- When possible, postpone making major life changes until spring or summer.

- Share experiences regarding SAD as a way to get information, understanding, validation, and support.

- If you are able, arrange for a vacation during the winter in a warm, sunny climate.

Mineral and Vitamin Deficiencies

The minerals calcium and magnesium are important in regulating transmission of nerve impulses in both your brain and skeletal muscles. Deficiencies of these minerals, due either to diet or poor intestinal absorption, can lead to chronic muscle tension and spasms, which can in turn make you feel anxious and uptight. You can easily identify deficiencies of these two minerals (and other essential minerals such as zinc and manganese) by having your doctor order a hair analysis test. This is the same test that is used to diagnose the heavy metal toxicities described earlier in this chapter. Even without the test, we recommend you take a daily dose of calcium (1000 to 1500 milligrams) and magnesium (500 to 1000 milligrmas), and you'll likely notice you feel more relaxed and sleep better. Many vitamin manufacturers combine these two minerals in a single capsule.

The B vitamins are also important to the maintenance and proper functioning of your nervous system. As mentioned in the next chapter, it's a good idea to take a B-50 complex capsule once or twice per day, especially if you're under stress. Higher doses of two B vitamins in particular can be helpful. Vitamin B_3 or niacin actually has functions in the brain similar to benzodiazepine tranquilizers such as Xanax and Klonopin (Larson 1999). Many people find supplementing in doses of 500 to 1000 milligrams per day can have a calming effect. The niacinamide form of B_3 is recommended over niacin, since the latter can cause flushing and tingling sensations. If you notice higher doses of niacinamide or niacin make you nauseous, stop for a day and cut your dose in half.   Vitamin B_5 or pantothenic acid is rapidly depleted when you are under stress. Supplementing with daily doses of 500 to 1000 milligrams will help strengthen your adrenals, increase your resilience to stress, and may ease allergy symptoms of all kinds.

Pyroluria

Between 20 to 40 percent of people with anxiety disorders have elevated levels of a group of body chemicals called kryptopyrroles, which are a useless byproduct of hemoglobin synthesis (Larson 1999). This condition is called pyroluria, and the problem is that it typically causes a depletion of the levels of Vitamin B_6 and zinc, which in turn can lead to a host of problems, including anxiety. Some of the symptoms of pyroluria include pale skin, sensitivity to sunlight, white marks on your fingernails (due to low zinc), depression, anxiety, and fatigue.

You can find out whether you're pyroluric by having your doctor order a test for kryptopyrroles (see the comprehensive Wellness Screening on pages 202–203 of this book). This condition can be treated by taking megadoses of Vitamin B_6 (200 millgrams twice per day) and zinc (25 millgrams twice per day), along with other daily supplements such as magnesium (500 millgrams), manganese gluconate (10 to 20 millgrams), pyridoxal-5-phosphate (50 to 100 millgrams), and niacinamide (500 millgrams). Since manganese and zinc compete with each other for absorption, it's best to take them at separate times. In consultation with your doctor, stay on this regimen for one month or until your symptoms improve.

Histamine Imbalances

Histamine is a chemical in your brain that helps to stimulate and regulate the release of neurotransmitters such as serotonin, norepinephrine, and dopamine. If the level of histamine is too low, dopamine levels in the brain can become elevated, leading to symptoms such as irritability and fatigue, and in extreme cases, paranoia and thought disorder. On the other hand, excessively high brain histamine levels have been associated with obsessions and compulsions. In a study done some time ago (Pfeiffer 1975), it was found that psychiatric patients with high histamine levels showed a significant reduction in obsessions and the need to engage in compulsive rituals when their histamine levels were brought down to normal levels. Not all people with obsessive-compulsive disorder have elevated histamine levels; however, having your doctor order a blood test for histamine might be worthwhile if obsessions and compulsions are a problem.

If test results show your histamine level to be too high, it can be treated by taking the amino acid methionine (1000 to 2000 millgrams per day) in divided doses on an empty stomach. A calcium-magnesium supplement (1000 millgrams calcium and 500 millgrams magnesium) will help methionine to work better. Stay with this regimen for one month, and then reduce the dose of methionine to 100 millgrams per day (methionine is a good antioxidant).

If, on the other hand, your histamine level is too low, it can be corrected by taking the amino acid histidine (a precursor for histamine), 500 to 1500 millgrams per day. Since histidine binds with zinc, it's important to take a zinc supplement (25 to 50 millgrams per day) along with it. Other supplements that assist with raising histamine levels include B_{12} (500 to 1000 micrograms per day) and folic acid (800 to 1600 micrograms per day). In consultation with your doctor, take histidine for two to three weeks and then stop. For more in-depth information about diagnosing and treating abnormal histamine levels, see the references by Pfeiffer and Larson at the end of this book.

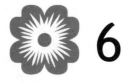 6

Natural Supplements for Anxiety

Certain supplements may offer a degree of relief from anxiety. In this chapter we'll give you a primer on the ones most commonly used to help with anxiety and stress reduction. These supplements include herbs, vitamins, amino acids, and hormones. Many of them have gained popularity in recent years, and it's likely that your local drugstore or health food store stocks them.

Some of the supplements discussed in this chapter have been used throughout history, and at present, many are used widely in Europe and the United States. You've probably heard of Saint-John's-wort and may know that calcium can have a calming effect. *GABA,* an amino acid associated with stress relief, is another supplement that's gotten a fair amount of press coverage in recent years.

It's important to remember that although you don't need a prescription for any of the supplements discussed in this chapter, when you ingest any of them (with the exception of vitamins) you are taking a form of medicine—and all medicines have risks. Some can aggravate preexisting conditions, some can interact with prescription medications in a way that causes dangerous or troublesome side effects, and many can engender side effects of their own. For example, SAM-e can intensify manic states in those with bipolar disorder and Saint-John's-wort should not be taken with MAO-inhibitor antidepressants.

This is why we recommend that you not try any of the herbal, amino acid, or hormonal supplements discussed in this chapter without first getting your doctor's approval. Ideally, you should consult a doctor who is trained in both conventional and complementary medicine, and he or she should monitor your treatment. Be sure to tell your doctor about any preexisting conditions you may have and any medications you're taking, and about the dosages and specific supplements you're considering. As we discuss each supplement, we'll point out the known adverse reactions and safety measures that we are aware of. You should remember, though, that these are *general* precautions and you are an individual with a unique medical profile. So additional concerns may come into play for you. If your doctor doesn't seem to be knowledgeable about supplements and their possible side effects and interactions with prescription medications, you can contact your local pharmacist or a holistically-oriented physician skilled in using supplements.

In trying any of the natural relaxers or antidepressants described below, *we recommend trying just one at a time to evaluate its effects*. Combining two or more natural supplements (for example, Saint-John's-wort, tryptophan, tyrosine, and SAMe for depression) in most cases is safe, but we recommend doing so in consultation with a knowledgeable doctor or health practitioner.

Herbs

In general, herbs work slower than prescription medications. If you're used to the rapid and intense effect of drugs like Xanax (alprazolam), you may have to be patient with the milder effect of herbs such as valerian. In many cases herbs can be as effective and have fewer side effects than standard medications like

Prozac. Several natural herbs can be used to help reduce anxiety. Kava and valerian are probably the best known and most widely used at present. Other herbs known for their relaxing effects include passionflower, skullcap, hops, gotu kola, and chamomile. Saint-John's-wort may have an anxiety-reducing effect for some people, but it is more widely used as a mild antidepressant. Each of these relaxing herbs can be taken individually or in combination with others. Most health food stores and many drugstores offer these herbs in three forms:

- the bulk herb, which can be boiled to make a tea;

- capsules; and

- liquid extracts, in which the herb is distilled and preserved in alcohol or glycerin, usually sold in a small bottle with a medicine dropper.

You might want to experiment with all three forms to see which you prefer.

KAVA

Kava (or kava kava) is a natural tranquilizer that has become quite popular in the United States in recent years. Many people feel that it is nearly as potent a relaxer as prescription tranquilizers such as Xanax. Polynesians have used kava for centuries, both in ceremonial rituals and as a social relaxer. Small doses produce a sense of well-being, while large doses can produce lethargy, drowsiness, and reduced muscle tension. In European countries such as Germany and Switzerland, kava was approved for treatment of insomnia and anxiety. Research in these countries has demonstrated kava can be effective in treating anxiety, worry, and insomnia (Cass and McNally 1998). It appears from limited research that kava may tone down the activity of the limbic system, particularly the *amygdala,* which is a brain center closely associated with anxiety. More specifically, kava appears to enhance the effects of the neurotransmitter GABA in the amygdala and other structures of the brain such as the *hippocampus* and *medulla oblongata*. Detailed neuro-physiological effects of kava are not known at this time.

Kava's principal advantage over tranquilizers such as Xanax or Klonopin (clonazepam) is that it's not addictive. It's also less likely to impair memory or aggravate depression in the way tranquilizers sometimes can. In fact, there is some evidence that it can improve concentration. Side effects are rare, though there are occasional reports of headache or a sense of being "washed out" following ingestion of high doses. Research, mostly in Europe to date, indicates that it is an effective treatment for mild to moderate anxiety (not panic attacks), insomnia, headache, muscle tension, and gastrointestinal spasm, and can even help relieve urinary tract infections (Cass and McNally 1998).

In buying kava, it is preferable to obtain a standardized extract with a specified percentage of *kavalactones,* the active ingredient. The percentage of kavalactones can vary from 30 to 70 percent. If you multiply the total number of milligrams of kava in each capsule or tablet by the percentage of kavalactones, you get the actual strength of the dose. For example, a 200 milligram capsule with 70 percent kavalactones would actually be a 140 milligram dose.

Most kava supplements at your health food store contain in the order of 50 to 70 milligrams of kavalactones per capsule. Taking three or four doses at this strength daily—up to 280 milligrams kavalactones divided into three or four doses—may be as effective as a tranquilizer. If you take this amount of kava all at once, it will function as a sedative and may help you to get to sleep at night.

At present there is little hard data on the effects of taking kava on a daily basis long-term, so it's advisable at this time not to use kava daily for more than six months. On an intermittent basis, however, you can use it indefinitely. If you are over age sixty-five, start with low doses of kava and increase the dose gradually. In general, it's not a good idea to use kava in combination with tranquilizers such as Xanax or Klonopin. While not dangerous, such a combination can produce grogginess and even disorientation. Especially if you are taking a moderate to high dose of Xanax or Klonopin (more than 1.5 milligrams per day), refrain from using kava. Avoid using kava if you are pregnant or breastfeeding, and use it with caution before driving or operating machinery.

An important caveat: In 2002 there were reports out of several European countries linking kava to severe liver damage. As a result, kava was banned in Germany, Italy, and England pending further investigation. There have been very few reports of problems with kava outside of Europe. Also, kava has been used for centuries in the South Pacific without known ill effects. In the United States, kava has not been taken off the shelves but is currently under investigation by the FDA.

Recent research has indicated a possible cause for the problem with kava in Europe. Traditionally, kava has been prepared using only the root of the plant and not the leaves and stems. In a research paper published in the journal *Phytochemistry,* researchers Klaus Dragull, Wesley Y. Yoshida, and Chung-shih Tang (2003) report they found an alkaloid called *pipermethystine* in the stem peelings and kava leaves. Pipermethystine is not found in the kava root. Several tests have indicated that pipermethystine has a strong negative effect on liver cell cultures. Evidence is also emerging that several of the kava producers in Europe used the leaves and stems of the plant, in addition to the root, in preparing their products, largely to save money and meet the enormous demand for kava that occurred in the past few years. If this evidence is borne out and further testing reveals that pipermethystine is definitely toxic to the liver, then there will be a reasonable explanation as to why some of the European brands of kava were associated with liver damage. Most forms of kava sold in the United States are derived solely from the root of the plant. Because kava has not yet been fully exonerated at the time of this book going to press, we would still recommend caution in using it at higher than the recommended doses or for longer than six months. Do not use kava if you have a history of liver problems or are using medications with known adverse effects on the liver. For further information on kava, see *Kava: Nature's Answer to Stress, Anxiety, and Insomnia,* by Hyla Cass and Terrence McNally.

VALERIAN

Valerian is an herbal tranquilizer and sedative that is widely used in Europe. In recent years it has gained popularity in the United States. Clinical studies, mostly in Europe, have found it to be as effective as tranquilizers in alleviating mild to moderate anxiety and insomnia (Davidson and Connor 2000). Yet it has fewer side effects and is nonaddictive.

Valerian is also not as likely as prescription tranquilizers to impair memory and concentration or cause lethargy and drowsiness. It will generally not cause a hangover the next day if used for sleep, though a few people have reported they are affected that way. In general, valerian can work well for mild to moderate anxiety, but may be less effective for more severe cases.

Derived from the plant *Valeriana officinalis,* valerian has numerous chemical constituents, including the essential oil, iridoids, and alkaloids. No one of these constituents is responsible for the sedative properties, and the overall impression is that all of the components work synergistically. So it's unlikely that a single component will be isolated and manufactured synthetically.

Valerian has a good reputation for promoting sleep. Numerous studies have shown that it can reduce the time it takes to get to sleep as well as improve the quality of sleep. If you try valerian for sleep and it doesn't seem to work, don't give up. Some studies indicate that it may take from two to three weeks of regular use for the herb to achieve its full benefit, whether you're taking it for insomnia or anxiety.

Valerian can be obtained at any health food store in three forms: capsules, liquid extract, or tea. In treating anxiety or insomnia, try each of these forms to see which you like best, following the instructions given on the bottle or package. Capsules are the most convenient, but some people swear by the efficacy of the tinctures and teas. Frequently you'll find valerian combined with other relaxing herbs such as passionflower, skullcap, hops, or chamomile. You may find these combinations to be more palatable or effective.

The effective dose for valerian ranges from 200 to 400 milligrams for anxiety relief during the day and 400 to 800 milligrams for help with sleeping at night. For sleep, it's best to take it about an hour before retiring. For mild to moderate anxiety during the day, you might take two or three doses in the 200 to 400 milligram range.

Be sure to buy a valerian product with sufficient potency. Generally, a statement on the bottle indicating that the product has been standardized to at least 0.5 percent of *valerenic acid* is an indication that it has reasonable potency. Also note if the bottle has an expiration date, as older products tend to lose potency. If the product contains other herbs or ingredients besides valerian, it should offer a complete listing of these along with the amount in each recommended dose. Avoid products that don't provide a full listing of ingredients.

As a general rule, you should avoid using valerian daily for more than six months. Long-term use at high doses has been associated with side effects such as headache, excitability, restlessness, agitation, and palpitations. You can use it two to three times per week, however, indefinitely. Also, valerian should not be taken together with benzodiazepine tranquilizers such as Xanax, Ativan (lorazepam), and Klonopin or sedatives such as Restoril (temazepam), Ambien (zolpidem), and Sonata (zaleplon). It can be combined with other herbs, such as kava, Saint-John's-wort, and especially hops or passionflower.

Long experience in Europe indicates valerian is an especially safe herb. Still, there are occasional reports of paradoxical reactions of increased anxiety, restlessness, or heart palpitations, possibly due to allergy. Stop using valerian or any other herb if it causes such reactions.

PASSIONFLOWER

Passionflower is a natural tranquilizer considered by many to be as effective as valerian. In higher doses it is often used to treat insomnia, as it both relieves nervous tension and relaxes muscles. It's available either in capsules or liquid extract at health food stores. Sometimes you'll find products that combine it with valerian or other relaxing herbs. It can also be obtained in a standardized extract containing 3 to 4 percent *isovitexin* (flavonoids). Generally, 200 to 600 milligrams is recommended for sleep, taken one hour before bedtime. Or you can take two or three 200 milligram doses throughout the day to relieve mild anxiety. The same precautions that apply to valerian apply to passionflower. In general, do not exceed doses recommended on the bottle.

HOPS

Hops is widely known as a component of beer. However, it's likely that the relaxing effects of beer have more to do with the alcohol content than the small amount of hops it contains. In Europe hops is widely used in a way similar to valerian and passionflower, as a treatment for anxiety, restlessness, and insomnia. Hops may be used alone, but more frequently it is combined with these other herbs, particularly valerian. The relaxing effect of hops is largely due to a specific chemical component: *dimethylvinyl carbinol.* In using hops, be sure to get it fresh. It tends to be unstable when exposed to light or air and loses its potency after a few months' storage.

GOTU KOLA

Gotu kola has been popular for thousands of years in India. It has a mildly relaxing effect and helps revitalize a weakened nervous system. It has also been found to help improve circulation and memory function and promote healing following childbirth. You can find it in most health food stores in capsules or extracts.

SAINT-JOHN'S-WORT

Saint-John's-wort (also called *hypericum*) has a long history of use. Hippocrates prescribed it for anxiety more than two thousand years ago. Currently it's used in the United States and Europe to treat mild to moderate depression and anxiety.

Although its primary impact seems to be on depression, Saint-John's-wort can reduce mild to moderate levels of anxiety as a secondary effect. It is probably not effective in relieving panic attacks, obsessive-compulsive disorder, or symptoms of post-traumatic stress disorder. European studies have found it to have antianxiety properties comparable to tranquilizers, although this finding has not yet been confirmed in the United States. Research has found evidence that Saint-John's-wort enhances the levels of all three neurotransmitters implicated in anxiety disorders: serotonin, norepinephrine, and dopamine (Bloomfield, Nordfors, and McWilliams 1996).

Saint-John's-wort is available in health food stores and many drugstores. Be sure to obtain brands that are standardized to contain 0.3 percent *hypericin,* the active ingredient. The standard dose is three 300 milligram capsules per day. Some people start out by taking two capsules per day and then raise the dose to three capsules daily. Taking Saint-John's-wort with a meal may limit any stomach upset that it causes. Unless directed by a qualified doctor, you shouldn't exceed 900 milligrams per day. Remember that Saint-John's-wort takes four to six weeks to reach therapeutic effectiveness.

Saint-John's-wort appears to have a good safety record. For some people, though, it can cause *photosensitivity,* an increased sensitivity to sunlight. Given this, you may want to limit your exposure to sunlight and use a sunscreen of SPF 30 or higher when taking it. Other side effects include stomach upset, dizziness, dry mouth, or allergic reactions. Also, the possibility that Saint-John's-wort may weaken the effects of oral contraceptives is currently being investigated. So far, it appears that the side effects associated with Saint-John's-wort are less than those caused by SSRI medications, such as Prozac, Zoloft, Paxil, or Celexa (citalopram). Unless instructed by your doctor, do not take Saint-John's-wort and SSRI medications together. If you're taking an MAO-inhibitor antidepressant, such as Nardil (phenelzine) or Parnate (tranylcypromine), do not take Saint-John's-wort. For more information on Saint-John's-wort, see

Hypericum & Depression by Harold Bloomfield, Mikael Nordfors, and Peter McWilliams.

SAM-e

S-adenosyl-methionine (abbreviated SAM-e, pronounced "Sammy") occurs naturally in the body. Widely popular in Europe for over a decade, it first became available in the United States in 1999 and is reported to have a significant antidepressant effect. SAM-e appears to work by increasing serotonin and dopamine activity in the brain. While healthy people manufacture enough of their own SAM-e, research has found that clinically depressed people are often deficient (Brown 1999). At this time information on the usefulness of SAM-e as an anxiety treatment is limited, but some people speculate that if SAM-e functions like an SSRI, it may have an antianxiety effect.

Side effects of SAM-e appear to be few, perhaps because it naturally occurs in the body. Some people report nausea or queasiness that goes away after a few days of taking it. SAM-e is unlike Saint-John's-wort and prescription antidepressants in that many people claim to feel its benefits within the first few days of use.

In addition to helping with depression, SAM-e may be helpful in the treatment of osteoarthritis and fibromyalgia. It appears to restore and maintain healthy joint function by contributing to the regeneration of cartilage. Also, it has potent antioxidant properties. The body uses it to help synthesize *glutathione,* an important antioxidant involved in protecting cells from free radical damage. It's believed that SAM-e can assist in detoxifying the body of substances such as alcohol, drugs, and environmental toxins.

SAM-e is available in most health food stores and drugstores in 200 milligram tablets. Enteric coated tablets are preferable because they are less likely to upset your stomach. The typical dose for depression is 800 to 1,200 milligrams per day, which should be taken at breakfast and lunch. Because it can cause slight nausea and gastrointestinal disturbances, some people choose to start with 200 milligrams twice per day and increase the dose to 400 milligrams twice per day after five days. People with bipolar disorder (manic depression) should know that SAM-e can aggravate manic states, and should avoid it unless their physician prescribes it for them.

Vitamins

Vitamins play a critical role in regulating the thousands of metabolic reactions that occur every moment in your body. While a majority of physicians, nutritionists, and health practitioners recommend supplementation, there is some disagreement over what constitutes appropriate doses.

Supplements can be helpful for several reasons. First, the average American eats a diet that is loaded with processed foods, which are vitamin-deficient. In addition, even people who eat fresh whole grains, fruit, and vegetables may not get sufficient amounts of minerals, due to the widespread depletion of minerals in soil that has been farmed for decades. Modern society imposes a variety of conditions that can deplete the body's store of vitamins. Stress, for example, can rob you of B vitamins, vitamin C, calcium, and magnesium. Smoking and drinking deplete certain B vitamins. Living in a polluted area can increase your need for antioxidant vitamins such as vitamin C, vitamin E, and selenium.

Fifty years ago, the U.S. Food and Nutrition Board established the *recommended daily allowance* (RDA) of vitamins needed by a healthy person. Advocates of supplementation say this recommended daily allowance constitutes the minimum amount of vitamins needed to prevent deficiency diseases such as scurvy and that the optimal amount is often significantly greater. Some nutritionists refer to these optimal doses as the *optimal daily allowance* (ODA).

In general, vitamins should be taken with meals. This is because stomach acids and enzymes produced while digesting food are necessary to help break down and assimilate vitamins. Vitamins taken in capsule form are usually easier to digest than tablets. Many health practitioners recommend taking vitamins along with digestive enzymes to improve their absorption and availability, especially if you're taking large numbers of vitamins with one or more meals.

B VITAMINS

B vitamins are a widely recognized casualty of stress. In difficult times, when you're feeling emotionally and psychologically tried, their levels can be depleted. Many people find that a daily dose of a high-potency vitamin B-complex increases their tolerance for stress and boosts their energy level. There are eleven B vitamins in all. Deficiencies in B_1, B_2, B_6, and B_{12} may contribute to anxiety, irritability, restlessness, and fatigue. Vitamin B_5 (pantothenic acid) supports the adrenal glands, whose proper functioning helps you to weather stress. Since the B vitamins tend to work synergistically, taking a B-complex supplement (which contains all eleven of the B vitamins) daily is probably optimal. The typical B-complex dosage is 50 to 100 milligrams of all eleven B vitamins daily. When under stress, some people find it helpful to take this dosage twice daily, and some take as much as 1,000 milligrams per day in a time-release form when they are experiencing pronounced stress. If taken on a long-term basis, vitamin B_6 should not exceed 100 milligrams daily.

Inositol

Inositol is a B vitamin that plays an important role in regulating the neurotransmitter serotonin within nerve cells. A well-controlled, double-blind study done by Israeli researchers in 1997 found that high doses of inositol (18 grams per day) were as effective as the SSRIs Prozac and Luvox in treating obsessive-compulsive disorder (Larson 1999).

Inositol has also been used to treat panic disorder and other anxiety disorders with good results. If you want to try inositol, obtain it in a powdered form (available at your health food store or on the Internet) and take 4 to 8 grams (about one teaspoon) three times per day with meals. Keep in mind that inositol is water soluble and safe, even at high doses.

VITAMIN C

Like B vitamins, vitamin C can become depleted in stressful times. It is widely believed that vitamin C enhances the immune system and aids healing from infection, injury, and some illnesses. Vitamin C also helps to support the adrenal glands. The typical dosage of vitamin C if you're dealing with anxiety difficulties is 1,000 milligrams in a time-release form two or three times a day. Some people double this in times of high stress. Be aware that repeated daily doses in excess of 8,000 milligrams have been associated with stomach complaints and even kidney stones in some people. Vitamin C in combination with bioflavonoids may offer greater benefit.

CALCIUM

Calcium can have a tranquilizing effect on the nervous system. Along with neurotransmitters, calcium is involved in the process of conveying signals across the synapses between nerve cells. Depletion of calcium can spur nerve cell overactivity, which may be one of the underlying physiological causes of anxiety. At least 1,000 milligrams of calcium per day is recommended. This can come in the form of either calcium-rich foods such as dairy products, eggs, and leafy vegetables; a supplement (chelates such as citrates or aspartates are preferred to calcium carbonate); or a combination of both. Calcium supplements should be combined with magnesium because these two minerals balance each other out and work in tandem. The ratio of calcium to magnesium should be either two-to-one or one-to-one. Liquid calcium-magnesium is also available at most health food stores and often produces an immediate relaxing effect.

Magnesium, taken on its own in a 500 milligram dose, may aid sleep. Also, soaking in a hot bath with one or two cups of Epsom salts is a great way to get magnesium into the body.

Uncovering Deficiencies Using Hair Analysis

If you suspect that you are deficient in calcium or other minerals, talk to your doctor about getting a hair analysis test. Deficiencies in a variety of minerals can be detected in a hair sample, and these deficiencies may suggest other conditions. For example, too little chromium may indicate a problem in carbohydrate metabolism and hypoglycemia. Too little cobalt can suggest an inadequate level of vitamin B_{12}. The hair analysis can also reveal excesses of toxic metals such as aluminum, lead, or mercury. High levels of mercury have been associated with anxiety disorders.

Amino Acids

Amino acids are the natural constituents of protein. In recent years they have become increasingly popular as complementary treatment for anxiety disorders and depression.

GAMMA AMINO BUTYRIC ACID

Gamma amino butyric acid (GABA) is a neurotransmitter that actually reduces excess neurotransmission in the brain. When used supplementally, it generally has a mildly tranquilizing effect, as only a small portion of what you take actually gets into the brain. It works by limiting excess activity in areas of the brain associated with anxiety. When GABA binds to the surface of certain neuronal receptor sites, the neurons become less active, which may tend to decrease anxiety. When taken with GABA, B-vitamins such as inositol, niacinamide, and vitamin B_6 enhance its ability to bind to receptor sites. Typically, GABA is taken in 200 to 750 milligram doses once or twice daily. Don't exceed 1,500 milligrams in a twenty-four-hour period except in consultation with your doctor. It's a good idea to take GABA on an empty stomach or with a carbohydrate snack like toast or crackers, which tends to enhance the sedative effect. Avoid taking GABA with protein, as this will tend to compete with the absorption of GABA.

GABA, in combination with the amino acids taurine and glycine, has been used to help people wean themselves off of benzodiazepine tranquilizers such as Xanax, Ativan, and Klonopin.

THEANINE

Theanine is a unique amino acid found almost exclusively in green tea. It promotes mental and physical relaxation without inducing drowsiness. Theanine not only has a relaxing effect but may also improve learning ability, heighten mental acuity, and reduce PMS symptoms. Preliminary evidence indicates that theanine helps in the formation of GABA. The recommended dose is 100 to 200 milligrams one to three times per day. Do not exceed 600 milligrams in one day. Theanine seems to work best as a natural relaxer during the day rather than as a sedative at night.

DL-PHENYLALANINE AND TYROSINE

DL-*phenylalanine* or *tyrosine* can be used to reduce symptoms of depression. They are particularly helpful if you experience low energy and lethargy associated with depression. We mention them here because many people with anxiety also suffer from depression. Both DL-phenylalanine and tyrosine increase the amount norepinephrine in the brain. A deficiency of norepinephrine has been associated with depression.

You should not take DL-phenylalanine or tyrosine if you are pregnant, if you have PKU (a disease requiring a phenylalanine-free diet), an active hyperthyroid condition, or if you are taking an MAO-inhibitor medication, such as Nardil or Parnate. Anyone with high blood pressure should avoid DL-phenylalanine or tyrosine unless instructed by his or her doctor. Preferably, they should be taken on an empty stomach, a half-hour before or two hours after a meal. The standard dose is 500 milligrams twice per day to start, increasing to 1,000 milligrams twice per day over three or four days. After one week, if there is no effect, the dosage can be raised to 3,000 milligrams per day. Do not exceed 3,000 milligrams daily unless directed by your physician. Unless you experience adverse reactions, try *either* DL-phenylalanine *or* tyrosine for two weeks. If one does not have an effect, try the other.

If you are severely depressed or have suicidal thoughts, you should not rely solely on these amino acids to resolve your illness. See a psychiatrist qualified to treat depression.

TRYPTOPHAN

The amino acid tryptophan is a natural precursor to the neurotransmitter serotonin. Serotonin is involved in regulating many body functions, including mood, sleep, appetite, and pain threshold. It produces a feeling of calmness and well-being, and deficiencies have been linked to anxiety.

Tryptophan is a potent antidepressant. A number of studies have found tryptophan to be as effective as prescription antidepressants and sedatives in relieving depression, insomnia, and generalized anxiety, as well as anger and irritability.

Tryptophan is available in two forms: 5-Hydroxytryptophan (5-HTP) and L-tryptophan. You can find 5-HTP in most health food stores. The recommended dose is 50 to 100 milligrams two to three times per day (or in a single combined dose at bedtime for insomnia), with or without food. L-tryptophan was widely used in the 1980s and then taken off the market in 1989 by the FDA. An impurity in the manufacturing process at a single company caused a rare blood disease that resulted in severe illness for several thousand people. In the mid-nineties, L-tryptophan was reintroduced in the United States under strict manufacturing standards and only by prescription. In the past few years, it has become available again without a prescription and can be obtained at some health food stores and over the Internet. Many people (including the senior author) find L-tryptophan to be more sedating than 5-HTP and so prefer it for insomnia. The recommended dose is 1000 to 2000 milligrams at bedtime, taken with a carbohydrate snack or fruit juice. If you take either 5-HTP or L-tryptophan, effectiveness can be improved by taking it along with Vitamin B_3 (niacinamide 100 to 500 milligrams) and Vitamin B_6 (100 milligrmas). If you are taking an SSRI, tricyclic, or MAO-inhibitor antidepressant, do not take either form of tryptophan except under the supervision of a physician.

For more in-depth information about the use of amino acids to treat anxiety and depression, see the books by Ross, Larson, or Slagles in the Further Reading/Resources section at the back of this book.

Omega-3 Fatty Acids

Omega-3 fatty acids, especially DHA and EPA, are important for brain and neurological health. Without sufficient levels of omega-3 fatty acids, nerve cell membranes are less fluid and may cause nerve cells to react slowly and misfire. Recent studies have found omega-3 supplementation to be helpful in diminishing symptoms of depression. The best source of omega-3 fatty acids is wild fish (especially salmon and sardines), meat, and fowl. Taking fish oil in liquid (two tablespoons per day) or capsules (two or three per day, or a combined dose of 1000 to 2000 milligrams per day) may help alleviate depression and mood instability. Oils should be stored in the freezer or refrigerator to protect them from damaging oxidation. Taking 400 IU daily of vitamin E (mixed tocopherol form) can also provide protection from oxidation.

Hormone Supplements

A variety of hormones are available to supplement presumed deficiencies. You've probably seen many of them at your local drugstore or health food store. Some may promote relaxation and aid sleep. Two of the most common are discussed below.

MELATONIN

Melatonin is a hormone secreted at night by the pineal gland to signal the brain that it is time to go to sleep. Supplemental melatonin can help you get to sleep as well as regulate sleep cycles. It is taken in doses from 0.5 to 3 milligrams. While many people find it useful, others say that they get no benefit from it and that it leaves them feeling groggy in the morning. If you experience no benefit or side effects from 2 to 3 milligrams, try lowering your dose to 0.5 milligram.

DHEA

Dehydroepiandrosterone (DHEA) is manufactured by the adrenal cortex and is used in the synthesis of other hormones in the body, including the sex hormones estrogen and testosterone. The ability to produce it declines with age. Many people report increased energy and sense of well-being, better ability to cope with stress, and improved mood and sleep after taking DHEA for a few weeks. The standard dose is 10 to 50 milligrams per day. Avoid taking it in higher doses, as some physicians believe that high doses can suppress the body's natural ability to make DHEA. Also, DHEA can be problematic for some women because they can convert it into testosterone. For this reason, women taking DHEA should take low doses (10 milligrams) or take a synthetic form that stays in the body as DHEA.

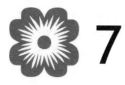 **7**

Meditation: A Journey to Inner Peace

Imagine for a moment that you're writing a letter to someone you've never met and want to give him or her a clear picture of yourself. You'd probably write things like *I like traveling and going to plays; I don't like sports; I love the summer, but hate the winter; I spend a lot of time cooking and dream of owning my own restaurant someday.* In other words, you would define yourself by what you like and dislike, what you want, and what you do.

Finding the Self beneath Your Identity

Meditation is paradoxical because it is a process of distancing yourself from these emotional and psychological attachments that seem to compose your identity and ultimately connecting to a deeper, more fundamental self—one that is not so easy to capture in language. When you meditate you become still and quiet enough to reconnect with your deepest inner self. This allows you to relinquish value judgments and achieve a better perspective on the thoughts, emotions, and desires that continuously cycle through your mind and body.

COMPASSION: MEDITATION'S GIFT

One of meditation's many benefits is that it helps you to develop a greater level of compassion toward yourself and others. Because bouts of anxiety often leave behind feelings of shame, guilt, and frustration, this is of particular value. Meditation helps you to witness your feelings without being consumed by them. It is an important tool not just for reducing symptoms but for minimizing anxiety's effect on your self-esteem.

Cultivating a more compassionate view of your conditioned thoughts and the emotional reactions they engender will help you establish a truce with them. To bring compassion into your self-observation is to begin to make peace with yourself and to view your shortcomings with a kinder eye.

If you are a perfectionist, you likely have a tendency to excoriate yourself for every minor flaw or mistake. You might want to take note of how much time you spend criticizing yourself, putting yourself down, or pushing and driving yourself to do what you don't really want to do. When you're not pushing or criticizing yourself, you may fall into a more passive stance of fear or of being a victim. Out of this fear, what-if thoughts can spring up and create more fear. When you see yourself as a victim, depression-inducing thoughts like *It's no use, It's hopeless,* or *It's a lost cause* can arise. Notice how much you criticize, scare, depress, or cajole yourself, and you'll learn quite a bit about your own mind.

Cultivating compassion in self-observation will help you shift to a more loving relationship with yourself. It allows you to move away from judgment, criticism, and even contempt, toward tolerance, acceptance, and love. Compassion depends on accepting yourself—and the rest of the world—as it is. Living with your limitations and embracing your humanness is something you can learn through the practice of meditation. For a more in-depth discussion of the role of compassion in meditation, see Jack Kornfield's book *A Path with Heart* (1993).

CREATING DISTANCE BETWEEN YOURSELF AND YOUR ANXIOUS THOUGHTS

Meditation practice is based, in part, on the belief that our automatic thoughts and emotional reactions to them are the source of all human suffering. Since ancient times meditation has been used as a means of transcending suffering and acquiring a healthy distance between ourselves and our thoughts. It is a process by which we step back and simply witness our thoughts without reacting to them. Sound familiar? In chapter 4 you learned some techniques for reflecting on and restructuring your thoughts before becoming emotionally embroiled in them. The cognitive behavioral techniques you learned in chapter 4 offered a psychological strategy for keeping anxiety symptoms from following thoughts. The meditation exercises in this chapter provide a more spiritual approach.

AWARENESS

Meditation is a path to expanded awareness. *Awareness* can be defined as a pure, unconditioned state of consciousness that everyone can experience. It exists "behind" or prior to the conditioned patterns of thinking and emotional reactivity we've learned over a lifetime. This awareness is always available to us, but much of the time it's obscured by the constant bustle of mental chatter and emotional reactions that inform our moment-to-moment experience.

Only when we become quiet and still, only when we allow ourselves to just be rather than striving to do anything, can this pristine awareness that precedes our thoughts and feelings reemerge.

To expand or enlarge awareness is simply to allow yourself to relax and settle into greater degrees of it. Awareness lies along a continuum, and it's possible to enter into it by degrees. According to ancient Eastern philosophy, your deepest inner awareness is a conduit to your higher power or God. At a deep level, your individual awareness flows into a greater universal awareness that has no limit, much as a drop of water is inseparable from the entire ocean. As you enlarge or deepen your personal awareness, you can begin to identify more with an infinite one. Remember that you don't have to do anything to enlarge your awareness; it is something that emerges naturally when you become still. When your awareness expands, you simply feel a deep sense of peace. Out of this inner peace there may arise other nonconditioned states such as unconditional love, wisdom, deep insight, and joy. In itself, this state of peace is nothing you need to develop.

Meditation allows you to expand your awareness to the point where it's larger than your fearful thoughts or emotional reactions. As soon as your awareness is larger than your fear, you are no longer swept up by the fear but are able to stand outside of it. You merely witness it. As you continue to practice meditation and enlarge your awareness, it becomes easier on an ongoing basis to observe the stream of thoughts and feelings that make up your experience without getting "stuck" or trapped in them.

Perhaps you think that becoming more observant of your thoughts and feelings would be a mistake, that you have such a cacophony of thoughts and such an ever-shifting stream of emotions that becoming more aware of them could only lead to greater division. It's important here to remember that we're talking about getting in touch with a deeper self, one that resides beyond the reactive thoughts and feelings that pull you away from it. When you do this you will be able to observe your thoughts and feelings without being pulled into their orbit. You will gain a greater sense of wholeness and a greater degree of freedom to live your life without getting mired in fear, anger, guilt, shame, grief, and other difficult emotions. With regular practice of meditation, you become more able to acknowledge your reactions, allow them to simply move through you, and then let go of them. When your mind is not riding the crest of every emotional wave, you develop a different and much healthier perspective on your feelings. In short, the greater your awareness, the less the impact of your conditioned thoughts and reactive feelings.

How to Just Be: Learning to Meditate

Learning to meditate is a four-part process. It involves cultivating right attitude, developing right technique, developing concentration, and maintaining your practice.

RIGHT ATTITUDE

The attitude or mindset that you bring to the practice of meditation has a profound impact on how much you will benefit from it. *Right attitude* is the optimal mental approach. It is the one that allows you to experience the full benefits of meditation, and cultivating it is an integral part of the overall practice of meditation. In *Full Catastrophe Living* (1990) and *Wherever You Go, There You Are* (1994), Jon Kabat-Zinn, a well-known teacher of meditation, discusses the following eight aspects of right attitude.

Beginner's mind. This is the mental state you occupy when you observe your immediate, ongoing experience without any judgments, preconceptions, or projections. In essence, it is perceiving a thought, a feeling, a situation, or a person as if for the first time. It's seeing and accepting things as they actually are in the present moment, not as they appear through the lens of your assumptions and judgments about them. Try this: The next time you're in the presence of someone familiar, consider seeing them as much as possible as they actually are, apart from your feelings, thoughts, projections, or judgments. Ask yourself, *How would I see this person if we had never met before?*

Nonstriving. In essence, almost everything you do in your day-to-day life is goal directed. You may not feel like you're on a quest when you get on the bus to go to work, but you do have a goal, and accomplishing it is essential for meeting other goals. You get on the bus so you can go to work; you go to work so you can pay your bills; you pay your bills so you can stay financially solvent; you stay financially solvent so you can have some long-term security . . . this chain of goals could circle the earth many times over. Meditation is one thing that is decidedly not goal driven. Although it takes effort to practice, meditation has no aim other than to just be. When you sit down to meditate, it's best to clear your mind of any goals—including goals that encompass the rewards of meditation. You are not trying to relax, to clear your mind, relieve stress, or reach enlightenment. The quality of your meditation should not be evaluated according to how close you come to these states. The only intention you bring to meditation is simply to *be,* to observe your here-and-now experience as it is. If you are tense, anxious, or in pain, don't strive to get rid of these sensations; instead, simply observe and be with them as best you can. Let them remain as they are. In doing so, you cease resisting or struggling with them.

Acceptance. This is the opposite of striving. As you learn to simply be with whatever you experience in the moment, you cultivate acceptance. Acceptance does not mean that you have to like what comes up (tension or pain, for example), it simply means you're willing to be with it without trying to push it away. You may be familiar with the saying "What you resist persists." As long as you resist or struggle with something, whether in meditation or life in general, you actually energize and magnify it. Acceptance allows the discomfort or problem to just be. While it may not go away, it becomes easier to deal with because you cease to struggle with or avoid it.

In life, acceptance does not mean that you resign yourself to the way things are and cease trying to change or grow. On the contrary, acceptance clears a space where you can reflect clearly and act appropriately since you are unfettered by your reactions to the difficulty. Sometimes, of course, it's necessary to go through a range of emotional reactions first—such as fear, anger, or grief—in order to get to acceptance.

In meditation practice, acceptance develops as you learn to embrace each moment as it comes without moving away from it. As you learn to do this, you discover that whatever was there for a given moment will change. More quickly, in fact, than if you tried to resist it.

Nonjudging. An important prerequisite for acceptance, as well as for beginner's mind, is nonjudging. When you pay attention to your ongoing experience through the day, you'll notice that you frequently judge both outer circumstances and your own moods and feelings. These judgments are based on your personal standards of what is "good" and "bad." If you doubt this, take just five minutes to notice how many things you judge in that short time. To practice meditation, it's important to learn not so much to stop judging as to allow yourself to gain some distance from the process. You can simply observe your inner judgments without reacting to them. Instead, you cultivate a suspension of any judgment, watching whatever comes up, including your own judging thoughts. You allow such thoughts to come and go, while continuing to witness whatever object you have selected as a focus for meditation.

Patience. This is a close cousin to acceptance and nonstriving. Patience means allowing things to unfold in their own natural time. It is letting your meditation practice develop—or stall—as it will, without rushing it.

Patience is needed to meditate for a half-hour to an hour every day. Patience is also required to persist with your meditation practice through the days or weeks when nothing particularly interesting happens. To be patient is to stop hurrying. This often means going against the grain of a fast-paced society, where rushing from one destination to another is the norm.

Sitting in meditation regularly will help you develop patience, as it will help you cultivate all of the characteristics described in this section. The attitudes that help you develop a meditation practice are the very same attitudes that are deepened by the practice itself.

Letting go. In India there is an efficient way to catch monkeys, recounts Jon Kabat-Zinn in his 1990 book *Full Catastrophe Living*. A hole just large enough for the monkey's hand is drilled in a coconut. The coconut is then secured to a tree by a wire. Then, a banana is placed inside the coconut. The monkey comes, puts his hand in the coconut, and grabs hold of the banana. The hole is small enough so the monkey can put his open hand in but cannot pull his closed fist out. All the monkey needs to do to be free is to let go of the banana, yet most monkeys don't let go.

We're a lot like these monkeys. We grab on to a particular thought or emotional state—sometimes one that is actually painful—and we don't let go. Cultivating the ability to let go is crucial to meditation practice, not to mention a less anxious life. When you hold on to any experience, whether pleasant or painful, you impede your ability to simply be present in the here and now without judgment or striving. Letting go is the natural consequence of a willingness to accept things as they are. If you find that prior to meditation, you have a hard time letting go of some concern, you can actually use your meditation as a means to witness the thoughts and feelings you're creating around the concern, including the thought of *holding on* itself. The more minutely you observe the specific thoughts and feelings you have created around a problem, the more quickly you'll be able to expand your awareness around that problem and let it go. When the concern is intensely charged emotionally, it's probably best to release your feelings by talking them out or writing in a journal before you sit down to meditate. Cultivating all of the attitudes described in this section will help with letting go.

Trust. Another important attitude to bring to meditation is a basic trust in yourself. This means you honor your own instincts, reactions, and feelings, regardless of what any authority or other person may think or say. You refrain from judging what comes up in your experience, and you believe in the inherent goodness of your essential self. The practice of meditation is about becoming more fully your own authentic self. Practicing awareness means taking responsibility for your own experience on a moment-to-moment basis. It's you and no one else who is responsible for your experience. To fully embrace that experience, you need to trust it. Trusting your own insights and wisdom helps you to develop compassion toward yourself as well as others.

Commitment and self-discipline. A strong commitment to work on yourself, along with the discipline to persevere and follow through with the process, is essential to establishing a meditation practice. While meditation is very simple in nature, it's not easy in practice. In a society that's oriented toward doing and accomplishing, learning to value and make time for "just being" on a regular basis requires a special commitment. Few of us have had the value of nonstriving instilled in us, and so learning to stop goal-directed activity, even for just thirty minutes a day, requires commitment and discipline. The commitment is similar to that required in athletic training. An athlete in training doesn't practice only when she feels like it, when there is time enough to fit it in, or when other people are available to keep her company. A serious athlete practices every day, whether or not she feels like it and even if it doesn't give her any immediate pleasure or benefit.

To establish a meditation practice, it's best to sit whether you feel like it or not, whether it's convenient or not. Try to sit six or seven days per week, for at least two months. If you find you're unable to sit that often at first, don't chastise yourself, just do your best. At the end of this time, if you've truly practiced regularly, the process will likely be enough of a habit (and sufficiently self-reinforcing) that you'll continue. The experience of meditation varies from session to session: sometimes it feels good, sometimes it seems ordinary, and other times you will find it difficult to meditate at all. Although the point is not to strive for anything, a long-term commitment to regular meditation practice can transform your life. Without changing anything that happens in your life, meditation can change your *relationship* to everything that happens, on a deep level. There may be no conscious aim of meditation practice itself, but the benefits that naturally follow from developing such a practice are profound.

RIGHT TECHNIQUE: THE NUTS AND BOLTS OF MEDITATION

There is a right technique in meditation. Learning it is crucial to your meditation practice. Probably the most important aspect is to sit in the right way, which means sitting upright with your back straight, either on the floor or in a chair. There seems to be a certain energetic alignment within the body that occurs when you sit up straight. It's not likely to happen when you're lying down or slouching, although lying down is fine for other forms of relaxation. It's also important to relax tight muscles before you meditate. Traditionally, the main purpose of yoga postures was to relax and energetically balance the body prior to meditating. Below are some guidelines for achieving right technique.

Find a quiet environment. Reduce external noise as much as possible. If you cannot be completely free of it, play a recording of soft, instrumental music or sounds from nature. The sound of ocean waves makes a good background.

Reduce muscle tension. If you're feeling tense, take some time (no more than ten minutes) to relax your muscles. Progressive muscle relaxation of your head, neck, and shoulders is often helpful (see chapter 1). The following sequence of head and neck exercises may also be helpful, and combining it with some PMR is probably optimal.

1. Slowly touch your chin to your chest three times.

2. Bend your head back to stretch the back of your neck three times.

3. Bend your head over to your right shoulder three times.

4. Bend your head over to your left shoulder three times.

5. Slowly rotate your head clockwise for three complete rotations.

6. Slowly rotate your head counterclockwise for three complete rotations.

Sit properly. You can sit properly either Eastern- or Western-style. To sit in the Eastern style, sit cross-legged on the floor with a cushion or pillow supporting your buttocks. Rest your hands on your thighs. Lean slightly forward so that some of your weight is supported by your thighs as well as your buttocks. To sit Western-style (preferred by most Americans), sit in a comfortable, straight-backed chair with your feet on the floor and legs uncrossed, hands on your thighs (palms down or up, whichever you prefer). In either position, keep your back and neck straight without straining to do so. Do not assume a tight, inflexible posture. If you need to scratch or move, do so. In general, do not lie down or support your head; this will tend to promote sleep.

Set aside twenty to thirty minutes for meditation. This is the optimal amount of time to spend meditating, although if you're a beginner, it's okay to start out with ten-minute sessions. You may wish to set a timer (within reach) or run a background tape that is twenty to thirty minutes long so that you'll know when you're done. If having a clock or watch available to look at makes you more comfortable, that's okay. After you have practiced twenty to thirty minutes per day for several weeks, you may wish to try meditating for periods of up to an hour.

Make it a practice to meditate every day. Even if you meditate for only five minutes, it's important to do it every day. Ideally, you should meditate twice daily, once after rising in the morning and once in the late afternoon or evening. One period of meditation per day is the minimum.

Don't meditate on a full stomach. Meditation is easier if you don't practice on a full stomach or when you're tired. If you are unable to meditate prior to a meal, wait at least a half-hour after eating to do so.

DEVELOPING CONCENTRATION: SELECT A FOCUS FOR YOUR ATTENTION

The final aspect of right technique is so important that it deserves special mention. In order to practice meditation, you'll need to work on developing your ability to concentrate or focus your mind. This will enable you to minimize the inevitable distractibility that visits your practice. There are forms of meditation, called *structured meditation,* that require steady focus on a particular object. Your own breathing cycle or a *mantra* (a repeated word or phrase) is commonly used as focal point. Other common objects of meditation include pictures, repetitive music, or a candle flame. *How to Meditate* by Lawrence LeShan (1974) offers more detailed information on structured meditation.

Mantra or breath-counting meditation exercises are useful when you first begin to practice meditation, because they will help you hone your concentration. Many people prefer practicing structured forms of meditation all of the time.

Other people prefer *unstructured* forms of meditation where the object of focus is simply the ongoing stream of thoughts and feelings that make up experience. The process of witnessing ongoing experience with acceptance and non-judgment is often referred to as "mindfulness."

During any form of meditation, it's generally helpful to close your eyes in order to reduce outside distractions. Some people, however, find they prefer to keep their eyes slightly open, just enough to see external objects indistinctly. This can reduce the tendency to be distracted by inner thoughts, feelings, and daydreams. Try this if you find that you are frequently distracted.

You are unlikely to be aware of just how distractible your mind is until you first sit down to meditate. In India it's said that the untrained mind acts like a crazed or drunken monkey. Structured meditation techniques are a way of focusing this kind of mind. Later, you may want to drop these forms and simply observe or witness (without judgment) whatever comes up in your ongoing experience.

When you do a structured meditation, it's important to concentrate on whatever you've chosen as your focal point, but not to force or strain yourself to do so. Proper meditation is a state of relaxed concentration. When thoughts, daydreams, or external stimuli distract you, don't try to hold on to them or to reject them too vigorously. Just allow them to come and go.

Exercise: Using a Mantra

1. Select a word or short phrase to focus on. This could be a Sanskrit mantra such as *Om Shanti, Sri Ram,* or *So-Hum,* or it could be a word or phrase that has significance within your personal belief system, such as *Let go, let God,* or *I am at peace.*

2. Silently repeat this word or phrase, ideally on each exhalation.

3. As any thoughts, reactions, or distractions come to mind, just let them pass over and through you, and gently bring your attention back to the repetitive word or phrase.

4. Continue this process for at least ten minutes.

Exercise: Counting Breaths

1. As you sit quietly, focus on the inflow and outflow of your breath in your chest or abdomen. Let yourself breathe slowly and evenly. Each time you breathe out, silently count the breath. You can

count up to ten and start over again, or keep counting as high as you like.

2. Each time your focus wanders, bring it back to your
   breathing and counting. If you get caught in an
   internal monologue or fantasy, don't worry about it
   or judge yourself. Just relax and return to the
   counting again.

3. When you lose track of the count, start over at one
   or at a round number like fifty or one hundred.

4. Continue this process for a minimum of ten
   minutes.

After practicing breath-counting meditation for a while, you
may want to let go of the counting and just witness the inflow
and outflow of your breathing.

MAINTAINING YOUR PRACTICE

Establishing a routine of just being is not easy. It takes moti-
vation, commitment, and self-discipline. Learning to meditate is
like learning anything else: it requires time, diligence, and regular practice to become proficient. This means not indulging your
I-don't-feel-like-it moods and meditating even when it may not
be convenient. Setting aside a regular time to practice for twenty
minutes to one hour each day makes this easier. The best times
are generally first thing in the morning upon waking or in the
evening, provided you are not too tired. Other possible times
would be before lunch or dinner. By setting aside a regular time,
you carve out a place for meditation in your life.

Besides personal commitment and self-discipline, there are
helpful external avenues of support. Probably the best is to find a
local class or group that meditates regularly. You may find such a
class at a local hospital or adult education program in your area. Or
there may be a freestanding meditation group within driving distance. You may even be able to find a teacher who can work with
you on a one-to-one basis. Programs in *transcendental meditation*

(TM), which is a form of meditation developed by Maharishi Mahesh Yogi, are offered in many areas. While TM teaches only mantra meditation, it's a good place to begin. Having the support of a group will help you to stay the course at those times when it seems hard to keep up your daily practice.

The Insight Meditation Society (IMS) offers meditation retreats in various places throughout the United States. A meditation retreat generally involves sitting in meditation for six to ten hours per day (with hourly breaks) for one to ten consecutive days, although a few go even longer. Doing a retreat is a powerful way to deepen your ongoing meditation practice, but it is generally not recommended for beginners. You can contact IMS by calling (978) 355-4378 or going to www.dharma.org.

 **8**

Mindful Exercise

Prana, ki, chi: do you recognize any of these words? Does *chi,* in particular, sound familiar? The closest English translation to each of them is "life force" or "vital energy." *Chi* is a traditional Chinese medicine term, and if it rang a bell, it may be because Chinese medicine is becoming more widely practiced in the West. *Prana* is a Sanskrit word that comes from the lexicon of Ayurvedic (traditional East Indian) medicine, and *ki* is used by practitioners of Japanese healing traditions. These schools of traditional medicine maintain that vital energy crisscrosses the body along channels, sometimes called *meridians,* and robust health—physical, mental, and spiritual—occurs only when its flow is unimpeded. Blockages of vital energy are thought to be the source of health woes. In fact, Chinese and East Indian medicine trace all disease back to various types and degrees of blockage in the flow of vital energy.

Exercises such as yoga, tai chi, and qi gong grew out of this belief, and practitioners of Eastern traditional medicine recommend them for a variety of health complaints and as preventative measures. Regular practice of them can help you to adopt a more serene, clear mindset, which in turn will likely make you less prone to anxiety.

Reuniting Body and Mind

Back in chapter 1 we recommended abdominal breathing and progressive muscle relaxation for calming anxiety. When you practice these methods, you engage in an exercise that incorporates both body and mind and helps them to act in unison. Remember Edmond Jacobson's point that when the body relaxes, the mind will follow? Just as PMR works on both the physical and mental planes, so do mindful exercises like yoga and tai chi. This is important, because anxiety can leave you feeling alienated from and insecure in your body. Although no external trauma has occurred, your body reacts as if it has, and over a period of time this can leave you feeling physically depleted, which in turn can affect your mental state, which affects your physical state, and so on. When you practice mindful exercise to bring body and mind into harmony, you begin to relax and feel more connected within yourself. As you experience yourself as more integrated and whole, you will also be less fearful.

One benefit of mindful exercise is increased clarity of thought. How can this help anxiety? Think back to chapter 4. Remember how you learned to respond rationally to fearful and unrealistic thoughts? When your mind is clear, your thoughts are more reasoned, and so your conclusions are more rational and thus less catastrophic. You are less likely to cling to unrealistically fearful predictions.

BEFORE YOU EMBARK ON A PROGRAM OF MINDFUL EXERCISE

It is always the best course of action to speak to your doctor or health practitioner before beginning a new exercise program. The mindful exercises discussed in this chapter are generally safe, yet there are some circumstances in which they should be avoided. Women who are pregnant, for example, should avoid qi gong. Because it can thin the blood and enhance circulation, qi gong should also be avoided if you have internal bleeding and after certain surgeries or injuries. As with everything, you should remember that you are an individual and "general" recommendations may not apply to you. This is why it is always wise to confer with your physician before undertaking a new exercise routine.

Yoga: Stretching toward Serenity

Actually, yoga involves a lot more than stretching. It encompasses a set of ethical precepts, dietary practices, a meditation regimen, breathing and concentration exercises, and the stretches or postures you're probably familiar with. In this chapter, when we talk about yoga, we mean the yoga postures. Dating back to Pantanjali, the second-century-B.C.E. philosopher who first formulated it, yoga is one of the oldest health practices in the world. The word *yoga* means to "yoke" or "unify." Its ultimate goal is to achieve unity of mind, body, and spirit. As you approximate this, it's believed, your mind and body will become stronger and you'll enjoy greater mental clarity and calmness.

Many people say that a regular practice of yoga helps to minimize anxiety symptoms. According to a survey conducted by the Yoga Biomedical Trust, 94 percent of the 838 patients who used yoga as part of their coping routine claimed some relief from symptoms (Goldberg 1993). Additional studies have suggested that a regular practice of yoga can be an effective tool for combating anxiety.

This is why yoga has been incorporated into some of the stress reduction, anxiety treatment, and anger management programs designed by mainstream clinicians. In addition, many people say that yoga simultaneously increases energy and vitality while calming the mind. At the very least, yoga is a great way to strengthen muscles and improve flexibility.

THE POSTURES

Along with the physical demands, yoga postures require you to focus your mind and adopt a particular attitude. Each posture embodies an attitude, whether it is one of surrender, as in certain forward-bending poses, or of strengthening the will, as in a backward-bending pose. As you do each posture, you mentally and physically embrace the attitude. By emphasizing certain postures and movements, you may be able to cultivate certain positive qualities or move through other negative, restrictive personality patterns. If you are interested in learning yoga, try one of the books or tapes in the list of resources at the back of this book. Also, many gyms, local YMCAs, and community colleges offer yoga classes.

ASANAS FOR ANXIETY

Asana is the formal word for a yoga pose. Certain asanas are particularly helpful for diminishing anxiety. The corpse pose, the cobra, and the child's pose all inspire calm and quietude. The corpse pose allows you to focus on total relaxation. When you do the cobra pose, you help to bring your mental focus inward, enabling you to concentrate and become less susceptible to distraction. As you might guess, the child's pose involves moving into a fetal position. The child's pose relaxes the whole body and directs the breath to the abdomen and pelvis, which helps to strengthen the muscles in those areas. All three poses are simple to do, and when you combine them with a program of deep relaxation, as discussed in chapter 1, they help to calm the nervous system. When practicing your relaxation routine, aim to keep your focus steadily inward, keep your eyes shut, and breathe from the abdomen, not the chest. (Note that a full yoga routine will involve many more poses than three.)

The Corpse Pose

Relaxation is not the only benefit that the corpse pose offers. It also aids circulation, improves the functioning of the nervous system, relaxes skeletal muscles, and relieves fatigue. Follow the directions below, practicing it for five to ten minutes.

1. Lie on your back with your arms spread out about twelve to eighteen inches from your side, palms open and up, and your feet spread about as wide as your shoulders. Place a folded blanket or towel underneath your head and neck.

2. Close your eyes and relax, breathing slowly and deeply from your abdomen, allowing the abdomen to expand with each inhalation and to fall with each exhalation.

The Child's Pose

In addition to promoting relaxation, the child's pose takes pressure off the intervertebral discs and helps to relieve lower back pain. This position should be held for no longer than five minutes.

1. Sit in a kneeling position with the tops of your feet on the floor and your buttocks resting on your heels. Keep your head, neck, and trunk straight.

2. Relax your arms and rest your hands on the floor, palms upward and fingers pointing behind you. Exhaling, slowly bend forward from the hips until your stomach and chest rest on your thighs and your forehead touches the floor in front of your knees.

3. As your body bends forward, slide your hands back behind you into a comfortable position with your arms straight. Do not lift your thighs or buttocks off your legs. Keep your arms close to your body, with palms up. It's okay to spread your knees slightly if this is more comfortable for you.

4. To release the pose, slowly lift your head and trunk, and return to a kneeling position.

The Cobra Pose

Not only does the cobra pose aid in relaxation, it also strengthens your shoulders, neck, and back; develops flexibility of the cervical vertebrae; and helps expand your chest. This pose should be held for five to ten seconds.

1. Lie on your stomach with your forehead resting on the floor, legs and feet together, with your body fully extended and relaxed.

2. Bend your elbows, keeping them close to the body, and place your hands palm down beside your chest, aligning your fingertips with your chest.

3. Inhaling from your abdomen, slowly begin to raise your head, allowing your chin to touch the floor as your head is stretched forward.

4. Slowly raise your shoulders and chest, look up, and bend your head back, arching your back up as far as possible without straining. It's best to use your chest and back muscles to raise yourself off the floor, instead of your arms and hands.

5. Exhaling, lower your body until your forehead rests on the floor.

Tai Chi: The Serpent and the Crane

Tai chi is an ancient form of movement intended to unite body and mind. It is said to have originated when a thirteenth-century Taoist monk in China watched a serpent and a crane in battle. As the crane attacked the snake, the snake would smoothly move its position, never allowing the crane to touch it. This scene inspired the monk to develop thirteen moves, which have been refined through the centuries. The graceful and fluid movements flow into each other and have names like "Fair Lady Works at

Shuttle" and "Stork Spreads Wings." Tai chi is practiced by millions of people in China, where it is often performed in the morning and in large groups. It is also popular throughout the rest of the world, and in recent years it has enjoyed an upswing in popularity in the United States. Many older people, in particular, find it of value because of its gentle, nonjarring movements.

Like other mindful exercises, tai chi aims to disperse energy blockages so that the regular flow of chi can be restored and brought back into balance. This is why it is sometimes a companion treatment to acupuncture. Tai chi masters claim that it also brings the opposing forces of *yin* and *yang* into equilibrium. Yang and yin represents polar opposite forces, such as earth and sky, active and passive, and male and female. Physically, all tai chi movements require use of opposites, such as left and right or extend and retreat.

Anyone can benefit from tai chi, regardless of age or fitness level. Because it requires regular, deep abdominal breathing, tai chi sharpens mental acuity and concentration. Tai chi improves balance because it relies on movements that alternate from side to side, and it provides a low-intensity aerobic workout. Tai chi lowers blood pressure and slows the heart rate; in fact, it may be even more effective than aerobic exercise in this regard. Also, tai chi opens the joints (especially the knees), strengthens the spine and lower back, and massages the internal organs. Students of tai chi enjoy many other benefits:

- wider range of motion

- greater strength

- increased flexibility

- improved muscle tone

- smoother coordination

- increased resilience to stress

- more energy

- better posture

- increased circulation

- a heightened sense of overall well-being

THE MOVEMENTS

If you've ever watched tai chi, you know how entrancing it can be, and you won't be surprised to hear that some people refer to it as "moving meditation." Each tai chi sequence is a set of incremental motions linked together, and performing a single sequence may take as long as twenty minutes. These movements are said to promote the flow of chi and harmonize body and mind. Many people report that as their mastery of these movements increases, they see a spillover effect in their everyday lives. They are better able to slow down, think clearly, and respond gracefully to everyday trials. Tai chi can also promote greater poise and concentration in regular physical movement. All in all, it's an excellent exercise for maintaining overall well-being and fostering serenity.

WHAT TO EXPECT IN A TAI CHI CLASS

If you're interested in trying tai chi, you can find classes offered at some health clubs as well as some martial arts schools (though tai chi is generally not used as a form of self-defense). Ideally, you should study with a tai chi teacher rather than learn from books or videos, although there are some excellent ones available. The movements can be challenging at first, and a good teacher will be sure to help you assume them correctly. You should wear flat shoes or socks and loose clothes.

The class, which usually lasts an hour, begins with the basic tai chi posture, in which you stand with your back straight, knees slightly bent, head slightly upturned, feet parallel and shoulder-width apart. Your arms should hang freely, and your shoulders should be slightly rounded. The *tantien* area, which is just below the navel, is where all movements should originate. In traditional Chinese medicine the tantien is the central home of the body's chi, and as you focus on it throughout the movements, your body awareness grows. When you master a basic tai chi movement, it can be completed in around ten minutes. While some people are quick to learn the basics, true mastery of tai chi can take a lifetime, even with the recommended daily practice. If you'd like to try tai chi but can't find classes in your area, see the Further Reading/Resources section at the back of the book for suggested videos and books.

Qi Gong: Meditation, Breathing, and Movement

Qi gong (pronounced "chee-gong") is a practice that dates back at least two thousand years. It integrates meditation, breathing exercises, and movements, all of which can be helpful in reducing anxiety. Like tai chi, qi gong is designed to resolve energy blockages that keep chi from flowing freely throughout the body. qi gong nourishes the body's internal organs by circulating vital energy. In turn, the free flow of this energy facilitates blood and lymph flow and even the flow of nerve impulses. qi gong continues to be a staple of Chinese health care, with an estimated 200 million Chinese practicing it daily. In the United States, qi gong is included in some hospital programs, adult education centers, and community centers.

Proponents of qi gong claim that it boosts the immune system because it increases the flow of lymphatic fluid, and that its ability to improve circulation helps to facilitate the elimination of toxic substances from the body. Qi gong can also reduce blood pressure, dilate the blood vessels, and heighten oxygenation of the tissues. Some advocates of qi gong believe that it enhances mood by regulating the function of various glands and the fluid surrounding the brain and spinal cord. While the effectiveness of qi gong has not yet been measured scientifically, most people concede that it can promote relaxation. Many conventional physicians admit that they have seen the health of their patients improve after they adopt a regular qi gong regimen.

WHAT TO EXPECT WHEN YOU TRY QI GONG

As with tai chi, it is best to start practicing qi gong by attending a class or consulting with a qualified qi gong practitioner. When you attend a class, you should wear flexible shoes and loose clothing. Abstain from eating or drinking (especially alcohol) for an hour and a half before the class begins. The instructor will begin by showing you simple practices. It is likely that he or she will recommend repeating each one six times and then reducing the number of repetitions as you become more proficient. He or she may ask you to stand with your legs apart and breathe deeply while making certain motions with your arms and legs. Although you should strive to follow the instructions and execute the movements as best you can, you don't have to be perfect. If you can't hold your breath or stay in a position as long as recommended, go for as long as you can.

Exercise: Circulating Vital Energy

The goal of this practice is to move chi along your meridians. You should repeat it three times, rubbing your palms together before each round.

1. Rub your hands together to build up heat. This helps to build chi.

2. As if washing your face, stroke your palms upward across your cheeks, eyes, and forehead.

3. Continue over the top and sides of your head, down the back of your neck, and along your shoulders to the shoulder joint.

4. Continue under your arms and down the sides of your ribcage.

5. At the lower edge of your ribcage, move your palms around to your back, across your buttocks, down

the backs and sides of your legs, and out the sides of your feet.

6. Trace up the inside of your feet and the inner surface of your legs, up the front side of your torso, and onto your face again, beginning the second round.

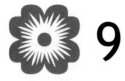 9

Keep It Simple

There is a difference between simplicity and austerity. An austere life is mired in want and deprivation; it is devoid of sensual pleasures and personal comforts. Whether or not you're dealing with anxiety, austere is the last thing we think your life should be! When we talk about a simple life, we mean a life full of activities, pursuits—and, yes, material items—that nurture your spirit and provide an outlet for fulfilling your values and your unique talents. We're talking about a life that is rich in valuable things and as free as possible of those financial and time commitments that deplete your resources without enriching you in some way. A life that is fettered with such commitments and crammed with superfluous material items fosters anxiety. A life that nurtures your talents, reflects your values, and bolsters your peace of mind invites serenity.

A Tale of Two Kitchens

Barbara and Paul have identical kitchens. They are both packed with the latest appliances and newest doodads for creating everything from the perfect breakfast to the ultimate cocktail party. In the pantry you'll find a deluxe mixer, a food processor, a juicer, a bread machine, a waffle iron, and an ice-cream maker. Besides the basics like measuring spoons and steak knives, the drawers bulge with handheld gadgets like lemon zesters and avocado scoops.

Paul is passionate about food and entertaining, and he spends more time in the kitchen than in any other room in the house. It is rare for a season to go by without a lavish party at his house, and he regularly puts his panoply of kitchen appliances to good use.

Barbara, on the other hand, doesn't really enjoy cooking and rarely has more than two people over at a time. She tends to buy things on impulse, and almost all of her kitchen items were spur-of-the-moment purchases that she used for a week or two and then retired to the pantry.

Where Barbara has clutter, Paul has a state-of-the-art workstation that he can use to indulge his passion and express his creativity. In this respect, Paul's life is simple because he has what he needs to do what he loves, and Barbara's is complicated because her space is crammed with extraneous items and her funds are wasted on things that don't reward her in the long run. What is unnecessary and onerous for one person can be vital to another. There is no precise formula for the simple life; ultimately, what constitutes a simple life for you depends on what you love and what you value.

One View of What It Means to Live a Simple Life

In his book *Voluntary Simplicity* (1993), Duane Elgin notes that people who choose a simple life tend to

- invest the time and energy freed up by simpler living in activities with their partner, children, and friends (for example, walking, making music together, sharing a meal, or camping)

- work on developing the full spectrum of their potential: physical (running, biking, hiking, and so on), emotional (learning the skills of intimacy and sharing feelings in important relationships), mental (engaging in lifelong learning by reading and taking classes), and spiritual (learning to move through life with a quiet mind and compassionate heart)

- feel an intimate connection with the earth and a reverence for nature

- feel a compassionate concern for the world's poor

- lower their overall level of personal consumption—buying less clothing, for example, with more attention to what is functional, durable, and aesthetic, and less concern with passing fads, fashions, and seasonal styles

- alter their patterns of consumption in favor of products that are durable, easy to repair, nonpolluting in their manufacture and use, energy efficient, functional, and aesthetic

- shift their diet away from highly processed foods, meat, and sugar, toward foods that are more natural, healthy, and simple

- reduce undue clutter and complexity by giving away or selling those possessions that are seldom used and could be used productively by others (clothing, books, furniture, appliances, tools, and so on)

- recycle metal, glass, and paper, and cut back on consumption of items that are wasteful of nonrenewable resources

- develop skills that contribute to greater self-reliance and reduce dependence upon experts to handle life's ordinary demands (basic carpentry, plumbing, and appliance repair)

- prefer smaller-scale, more human-sized living and working environments that foster a sense of community, face-to-face contact, and mutual caring

- participate in holistic health-care practices that emphasize preventative medicine and the healing powers of the body when assisted by the mind

- change transportation modes in favor of public transit, carpooling, smaller and more fuel-efficient autos, living closer to work, riding a bike, and walking

Some Ways to Simplify

Below are a few suggestions for simplifying your life. Some are changes you can make immediately, while others require more time and effort. Remember that the goal of the simple life is to free yourself from those commitments that deplete your time, energy, and money without meeting your essential needs or sustaining your spirit.

Downsize your space and expand your comfort. Smaller living quarters offer a couple of benefits. First, it's just not possible to accumulate a prodigal number of possessions without sufficient room for them. Also, a smaller space takes less time to clean and maintain as well as being less expensive. In *The 50 Best Ways to Simplify Your Life* (2001), Heather Garnos Mitchener and Patrick Fanning encourage readers to think about what an ideal simple home would mean for them. They suggest the following exercise: Close your eyes and visualize the elements you need for your ideal simple home. When you have a clear picture, put your ideas down on paper. Be as general or as specific as you like.

Imagine an organized linen closet, a quiet corner with a comfy chair, a spalike bathroom. Use your "simple home wish list" to start figuring out what steps you can realistically take to create such a simple home. Ask yourself where you want to spend the most resources, what can be accomplished with time and ingenuity rather than money, and whose help you might need to make these changes.

Cut clutter. We live in a time of unprecedented abundance. It's very easy to accumulate stuff that has no real value or use to us and only creates clutter—and anxiety. Mitchener and Fanning suggest cutting clutter by making a commitment to rein in your household purchasing, at least until you know what you already have squirreled away in the nooks and crannies of your home. Most likely you'll be surprised by how much stuff you own that you've entirely forgotten about. If you've forgotten about it for a year or more, do you really need it?

Make a change to right livelihood. *Right livelihood* is a Buddhist ideal that can be summed up in the 1960s admonition to be "part of the solution, not part of the problem." Right livelihood means working at a job that is consistent with your values and engages you on a personal level. It simplifies your life by giving you a sense of mission. When your work matches your values, your self-esteem rises and you can more easily weather complications, disappointment, and stress. Shifting to right livelihood may require time, risk, and effort. It may take one to two years to gain the retraining or retooling you need to begin a new career. Then you may have to endure some time at an entry-level position before your new line of work meets your financial needs. The time, effort, and disruption are usually well worth it.

Reduce your commute. Reducing or eliminating your commute is one of the most significant changes you can make to simplify your life. It doesn't take much reflection to see the extent to which negotiating rush hour traffic on a daily basis can add to stress. Moving closer to where you work or choosing to live and work in a smaller town can help reduce your commute. At the very least, if you have to commute over a long distance, you can try to arrange for flexible hours (to avoid rush hour) or have a comfortable car with a stereo. At this time, nearly 15 percent of Americans work out of their homes, and the number is rising. If you can figure out a consulting service or computer-based job you can do out of your home, you can join them.

Reduce your exposure to TV. How much time during the day do you spend in front of a screen? If you're like most Americans, your household has at least two TVs, each offering a staggering number of programs to choose from, and at least one computer with Internet access to millions of Web sites. Granted, there are many good programs on TV, and the Internet is a wonderful tool for communicating information. The concern is with the sheer complexity of having so many options, all of which involve a passive stance of either witnessing entertainment or absorbing information. While life in front of the screen can be a distraction from anxiety, it can also be a hindrance to rebuilding a deeper connection with nature, others, or yourself. If anxiety is aggravated by too much stimulation and an experience of disconnection, then it seems that spending time in front of the screen might be done in moderation.

Live close to nature. Anxiety states are often associated with feelings of disembodiment. Being ungrounded and out of touch with your feelings and physical body is especially evident in the sensations of depersonalization or derealization (the feeling of being "not all there") that can accompany acute anxiety or panic. This disconnection can be aggravated in situations that involve being literally disconnected from the earth, such as riding in a car, being high up in a tall building, or flying. It may also be aggravated in situations where you are bombarded with so many stimuli that your awareness is scattered, such as at a grocery store, shopping mall, or social gathering.

Taking a walk in the woods or a park is a simple act that can help reverse the tendency to feel disembodied. Being in close proximity to the earth—its sights, sounds, smells, and energies— can help you to remain more easily connected with yourself. Choosing to live in such a setting, if possible, allows you to reestablish the ongoing connection with the earth that much of modern civilization seems to have lost.

Tame the telephone. There are people who feel they should answer the phone virtually every time it rings, regardless of the time of day or the mood they're in at the time. Whether the caller is a creditor, a sales solicitation, or a cantankerous relative, some people feel it is an almost sacred obligation to answer every call. Remember that answering the telephone is optional. You can let your voice mail or answering machine pick up, and return the call when you are ready to give the caller your full attention. If you're engaged in a project or activity that you find rewarding, there's no need to drop it to take a call that does not require your immediate attention.

Delegate menial chores. Delegating even one activity you don't like to do, such as housecleaning or yard work, can make a difference in the sense of ease you bring to your day-to-day life. Is there something your children could learn to do just about as well as you? Perhaps you can allow other family members to help with the cooking, dishwashing, yard upkeep, or housecleaning. In *The 50 Best Ways to Simplify Your Life,* Mitchener and Fanning give some hints for deciding what should be hired out. They say to start by making a list of routine chores around the house and yard. Next, write down the big jobs that only have to be done a few times a year. Take an unsparing look at your list. Which routine chores do you chronically avoid? Do they build up to the point where you become anxious just thinking about them? Would getting those things done by someone else take some of the pressure off of you? Think about the big tasks like spring cleaning or window washing. Do you keep postponing these tasks year after year? If so, think about hiring someone to do them. If finances are an issue, perhaps you have some skill or item that you can use to barter with. Maybe there are teenagers or young people around who can use a part-time or temporary job.

Learn to say no. *No* is not a dirty word. Many people pride themselves on always being able to accommodate the needs and wants of their friends, family, and coworkers. The problem is that the end result of this consistent "helpfulness" is exhaustion. You can become so busy taking care of others' needs that you have no time or energy to take care of your own. When someone asks you for your time, effort, or anything else, think about whether it serves both your highest interest and the other person's highest interest to respond with a yes.

Slow the flow of information. More than ever, information is a source of clutter. Junk mail, catalogs, magazines, and newspapers can pile up until you have a mountain worthy of Sir Edmund Hillary. It's good to keep in mind that the information we expose ourselves to should be in line with our interests. Whether you're interested in local politics, news from countries that don't get much attention in the press, or perhaps the activities of Congress, you should filter out the information that you care about and let the rest flow by. They also suggest unsubscribing to the e-mail newsletters that you don't have the time or interest to read on a regular basis and dumping any subscriptions to magazines or newspapers that you don't read or enjoy.

There are a number of concrete steps you can take to stem the flow of information. For example, you can reduce the amount of junk mail you receive by writing to Stop the Mail at P.O. Box 9008, Farmingdale NY 11735. Request that your name not be sold to mailing list companies, and you will likely reduce your junk mail by up to 75 percent.

Exercise: Simplify-Your-Life Questionnaire

Now it's your turn. Take some time to think about ways in which you might simplify your life. Answer the following questions on a separate sheet of paper:

1. On a 1-to-10 scale, with 1 representing a high degree of simplicity and 10 representing a high degree of complexity, where would you rate your own lifestyle at present?

2. Have you made any changes in your living arrangements in the past year toward simplicity? If so, what changes?

3. What changes toward simplifying your life would you like to make in general?

4. What changes toward simplifying your life are you *willing* to make in the next year?

Exercise: Checklist for Living Simply

Review the following simplification strategies and check off the ones you would be willing to try or initiate in the next two months. Underline those you'd like to do in the next year or two.

- reduce the clutter in your home

- move to a smaller house

- move to a smaller town

- move close to shopping resources so you can do all of your errands quickly

- buy less clothing, with attention to what is functional, durable, and aesthetic rather than trendy

- drive a simple, fuel-efficient car

- reduce your dependence on TV

- reduce dependence on outside entertainment (movies, plays, theater, concerts, nightclubs)

- reduce (or eliminate) magazine subscriptions

- stop newspaper delivery

- stop junk mail

- stop answering the phone every time it rings

- reduce your commute (if possible, walk or ride your bike to work)

- work where you live

- tell everyone but your immediate family you no longer do Christmas gifts (or cards, for that matter)

- take one suitcase if you vacation, and pack only essential clothes

- take your vacation near or at home

- reduce your consumption to avoid luxury or designer items; favor products that are durable, easy to repair, and nonpolluting

- take steps to get out of debt

- keep only one credit card

- consolidate your bank accounts

- delegate busywork like yard work, housecleaning, and tax preparation

- simplify your eating habits to include whole, unprocessed foods

- buy groceries less often, in bulk

- make water your drink of choice

- pack your own lunch

- learn to say no

- stop trying to change people

- stop trying to please people—be yourself

- dispose of all personal possessions you don't really need

❑ do what you truly want for a living

❑ work less and spend more time with your loved ones

Some of these changes can be made quickly; others involve a process. It may take a year or two, for example, to arrange your life so that you're doing something you truly enjoy for a living. To dispose of unnecessary possessions, put aside things you think you won't need for a year in a locked closet or storage compartment. At the end of the year, if you've not given them any thought throughout the entire time, let them go. Learning to say no or to stop always trying to please other people requires that you develop assertiveness skills, which you can acquire through classes, workshops, counseling, and books. Remember that simplifying your life is a process of bringing your activities, work, and pursuits into closer alignment with your spirit.

 **10**

Embracing Spirituality

Spirituality, at least as we define it, is not synonymous with religion, and you don't have to hold to any particular religious doctrine in order to explore and deepen the spiritual dimension of your life. For our purposes, cultivating spirituality means developing a greater awareness of something that is larger than your personality and your day-to-day existence. Making a spiritual connection means moving beyond the ordinary realities of life to join with a higher power. Whether you decide to label this higher power *God* or *love* or *the universe* is, in this context, unimportant. What counts is that you cultivate a stronger sense of your interconnectedness with it.

When you deepen your spiritual awareness, you come to appreciate the inherent uniqueness of your purpose for being here on earth. The gravity of your daily worries and fears diminishes when seen through a wider spiritual lens. Anxiety and the what-if scenarios that often drive it can seem inconsequential after you've developed a stronger spiritual grounding.

How Spirituality Can Bring Calmness

While spirituality is by no means a replacement for conventional anxiety treatment, it's a powerful element of any complementary plan. Traveling on a spiritual path can lead to changes in your perceptions, attitudes, and beliefs that can have a significant impact on your anxiety.

Hope for recovery. Anyone who's struggled with anxiety knows that the path of recovery is not a straightforward or uniformly even one. Setbacks, frustration, and discouragement are a part of recovery, and it can sometimes seem like fear will be a constant burden. Spirituality can bring hope: hope that your distress will subside and that the future will offer many things besides fear. To be involved with some form of spirituality is to regularly experience inspiration, which can motivate you to persist in your efforts toward healing. The word *inspiration* literally means "in-spiriting." Spirituality doesn't take the place of learning and practicing the tried-and-true skills for symptom control, but it does provide the impetus to persist even when the road gets rocky.

A way to handle the tougher challenges. We are fortunate to live in the age we do. Good treatments for many anxiety disorders are readily available. Yet, some of the most intense cases of anxiety conditions like post-traumatic stress disorder or severe obsessive-compulsive disorder may improve only modestly with standard treatments like cognitive behavioral therapy and medication. In these situations spirituality may have much to offer. Following the twelve-step model and turning over a problem to a higher power has helped many people overcome challenges that seemed insurmountable. So has the process of visualizing or affirming your ultimate recovery, despite any difficulties you currently face. Deepening your spirituality may not translate into total freedom from your symptoms, but it can give you a new perspective on them that offers a comparable degree of relief. You can learn to live more peacefully with a problem so that it is a manageable fact of life rather than a chronic catastrophe. Developing greater inner peace, strength, and faith can lead you to accept your difficulties with equanimity. Acceptance is not the same as resignation or fatalism. When you work with a problem on a spiritual plane, you use it as a way to deepen your relationship with your higher power and to evolve as a human being. Your anxiety can then become a vehicle rather than a roadblock.

Security in volatile times. Anxiety is the antithesis of security. It is often triggered by a sense of being exposed to catastrophe, and it can leave you feeling as though you are controlled by your fear. Spirituality offers the precious gift of inner security and safety, and this can go a long way in easing anxiety. When you connect with your higher power, you gain security through the conviction that you are not all alone in the universe, even at those times when you feel alienated from others or battered by your anxiety. You feel increasingly safe as you come to believe that there is a source you can always turn to in times of difficulty. There is much security to be gained through the understanding that there is no problem or difficulty, however great, that cannot be resolved with the help of your higher power.

Peace of mind. Peace of mind is the result of feeling a deep, abiding sense of security and safety. The more reliance and trust you develop in your higher power, the easier it is to deal with the inevitable challenges life brings without worry or fear. It's not that you give up your will to such a power; rather, you learn that you can let go and rely on your higher power when you feel stuck in a problem. Learning how to let go when solutions aren't immediately apparent can help to reduce worry and anxiety. Peace of mind can be defined as the absence of worry.

Distance from automatic emotional reactions. Spiritual practices, particularly meditation, can help you to become more in touch with your fundamental self—the one that hasn't been conditioned by a lifetime of experiences and emotions. This is a deep inner state of consciousness, beyond ego, that is always still and at peace no matter what melodramas you may be caught up with in your day-to-day life. Moving into your unconditioned self is like reaching a calm oasis that lies outside the boundaries of anxiety. You can gain access to this state with time and practice. Meditation, quiet time devoted to inspirational reading, guided visualizations, inspirational music, or physical disciplines such as yoga or tai chi are all paths to it.

Release from your need to control. Worry arises when you fixate on circumstances that you can't fully control. Worrying offers you the illusion of control. If you worry about something enough, you feel somehow that you'll be better prepared for the disaster when it strikes; you won't be caught off guard. You imagine that if you were to stop worrying, you would give up control. Spiritual growth, regardless of the tradition or approach you choose, encourages the cultivation of a willingness to surrender control. Without relinquishing responsibility, you learn to allow your higher power to have some influence in determining the outcome of situations beyond your control. The phrase *Let go and let God* affirms this kind of attitude. This aspect of spiritual growth can have a direct impact on anxiety reduction.

Greater love and compassion toward yourself. As you cultivate a connection with your higher power, you strengthen the bonds between yourself and all creation. You remember that like the birds, stars, and trees, you are part of the universe. You also become more likely to view the universe as benign and supportive and to see yourself as good, lovable, and worthy of respect by virtue of being part of the universe. We treat our pets with respect and love just for being who they are, yet we often fail to do so with ourselves. However you behave, whatever choices you make, you are still inherently good and worthwhile. Your own judgments of yourself, however negative, do not ultimately count if you are a creation of the universe as much as everything else. It is, of course, a mistake to assume that this type of reasoning can be used to justify ignorant or unethical behavior. It's important to keep in mind the distinction between how a person behaves and who the person is in essence.

Freedom from perfectionism. If you believe that you are inherently valuable, you're more likely to avoid the pitfall of perfectionism.

When self-worth indeed comes from *self* rather than outward achievements, there is no need to obsess about meeting unrealistic standards, whether they are imposed by you or by the society around you. Of course, setting goals, building as full a life as possible, and striving to do your personal best can provide structure and make you feel more engaged in life. The problem comes not from striving but from measuring your value by your ability to achieve your goals—and achieve them completely. When you fully apprehend that your value comes from within, you are more likely to enjoy your pursuit of fulfillment and accomplishment rather than feeling enslaved to it.

Unconditional love. Connecting with your higher power means experiencing unconditional love. The source of all creation is itself an expression of pure love. Such love differs from romantic love or ordinary friendship. It is compassion and caring that does not hinge on what you or others say, do, or feel. It is free of judgment, and as you receive it you will find yourself giving it more willingly. You will likely feel your heart opening more readily to other people and their concerns. You'll be more likely to see them without the shadow of judgment and to resist making comparisons between other people and yourself or anyone else. Unconditional love fosters a sense of security, which is a natural antidote to fear.

Finding Your Own Spirituality

One thousand years ago, the medieval theologian St. Anselm argued that any concept of God is a contradiction, because God is infinite and anything that is truly infinite must be greater than any concept we can grasp. Nonetheless, attempting to comprehend the divine is a fundamental human compulsion. To think about or discuss a higher power, it seems necessary to have some concept of what God is, even if it's unavoidably incomplete.

What is your concept of and relationship to a higher power? The following questions are designed to help you formulate your thoughts about the answer to this question. Write your answers on a separate sheet of paper.

1. What does the idea of God or a higher power mean to you personally?

2. Describe the attributes defining your notion of God, spirit, or a higher power. When you think about the nature of God, what ideas and images come to mind? Is God personal or impersonal? Close or distant? Inside or outside?

3. Do you experience a personal, conscious connection with your higher power? How have you experienced this connection?

4. What obstacles do you feel interfere with your acceptance or experience of a higher power?

5. What would you hope to gain by developing or deepening your connection with a higher power?

FOSTERING CONNECTION BETWEEN YOU AND YOUR HIGHER POWER

Cultivating a relationship with your higher power is in some ways similar to developing a relationship with another person. The more time and energy you dedicate to it, the closer and richer the relationship becomes. If you're willing to give your relationship to your higher power more time and effort, it will become an important part of your daily life. Here are some of the ways people integrate spirituality into their everyday lives.

Prayer. Prayer is a way of actively communicating with your higher power, usually in the form of a request. Sometimes you may ask for a particular quality, such as strength, peace, or clarity. Other times you may ask your higher power simply to be present in a particular situation. Or you may relinquish a problem to God without asking for anything in particular.

Meditation. When you meditate you become quiet and still enough to get in touch with a deeper part of your inner being, one that is nonreactive, beyond conditioning, and ultimately in tune with your higher power. Meditation helps you to disentangle from emotions and thoughts that limit you, so that you can witness rather than react to them. For thousands of years, meditation has been a way to still the mind and directly access the kingdom of heaven within.

Reading spiritual literature. Reading uplifting spiritual books (or listening to tapes) is a wonderful way to move away from worry or a negative mindset. Whether you choose traditional sacred texts or contemporary books, reading spiritual literature can be uplifting, comforting, and enlightening.

Spiritual fellowship. Recognizing the sacred in the presence of others is a common and powerful way to renew your connection with God. This can happen through church attendance, spiritual classes and workshops, or sacred rituals.

Compassionate service. Volunteering to serve others or carrying out simple acts of kindness can bring spiritual rewards and make your life much richer.

Rituals and practices. Engaging in rituals and practices that grow out of traditional religions or modern spiritual movements can deepen your connection to a higher power. These include

- attending twelve-step groups and working the steps to overcome specific addictions

- listening to sacred music, either classical or modern

- sacred singing or chanting

- sacred dancing, for example, Sufi dancing

- practicing guided visualizations

- working with spiritual affirmations

- attending classes or workshops on religious topics

Exercise: Your Spiritual Practices

Write your answers to the following questions on a separate sheet of paper.

1. Do you pray? How often? With what effect? Do you believe your prayers have been heard or answered?

2. Do you meditate? How often? For how long? With what effect?

3. Do you read religious or inspirational teachings? How often? With what effect? What teachings have influenced you the most?

4. Do you engage in any other spiritual practices, such as chanting, rituals, singing, dancing, or vision quests? How often? With what effect?

5. Are you involved with a church, center, or other spiritually based group of people? How often are you in contact with this group? What do you get out of it?

6. Which of the above activities would you be willing, in the next month, to give more of your time?

Ideas to Ponder

Embracing the spiritual side of life can help you to reframe the way you perceive your own difficulties with fear or anxiety. As you delve deeper into your spirituality, you will likely find insights into the meaning of your problem with anxiety as well as how to go about healing it. The following ideas can help you to think about your own spiritual views. Give yourself time to reflect on, accept, reject, or just grapple with these ideas.

Life is a school. The primary meaning and purpose of life is to learn. Life is a classroom for growth in consciousness. The tasks and challenges that arise in life—and your response to them—do not have eternal repercussions, yet they are not devoid of meaning. They are like lessons in a school, lessons to which you apply yourself and which you try to master as best you can. Each lesson is repeated until it's mastered. As you master old lessons, new ones are put before you. In essence, life on earth is a place where you learn and grow.

Adversity is the springboard of growth. Challenges to our happiness and contentment are not random, capricious acts of fate. In the larger scheme of things, everything happens for a purpose. If you accept the idea that life is a classroom, then the adversity and difficulties that come into your life may be seen as part of the curriculum. This is a very different point of view from one that sees life's misfortunes as random quirks of fate. The latter perspective leads to a sense of victimization. You can end up feeling powerless in an erratic world that seems to blindly dispense fortune and hardship.

The view proposed here is that the difficulties of your life are lessons to promote greater wisdom, compassion, love, and other positive qualities. The greater the difficulty, the greater the potential for learning and growth. If you accept this idea, then your next question may well be *Who establishes the curriculum and assigns the lessons?* Many of us ask this question in one form or another when life deals us an unexpected blow. It's not unreasonable, after all, to look at our own and other people's difficulties and ask *How could a loving God permit this?* Of course, there is no easy answer to this question. None of us can fully understand how our life lessons are administered and assigned, though different spiritual traditions have different views on this matter. We have to struggle with the challenges life brings without fully understanding why. Yet, if you accept the notion that the purpose of life is for us to grow in wisdom, consciousness, and compassion, then you can probably see why some of the lessons need to be difficult. This may not be an altogether consoling view, but it at least makes some sense out of the tailspins into which life occasionally throws us.

Personal limitations are a source of growth. Our innate shortcomings inspire us to push toward our ultimate potential. Think for a moment about your anxiety. You may ask why anyone should have to deal with a difficult condition such as panic disorder, agoraphobia, social phobia, or obsessive-compulsive disorder for even a few months, let alone a number of years. Perhaps you have utilized all of the best treatments (including medication if necessary) and have experienced a significant and genuine recovery. In many cases, a full recovery from an anxiety disorder is possible. Suppose, however, that you have received all the best treatments, worked very hard over a long period of time, and have still not achieved full remission. Is that a reason for you to think of yourself as a failure? A reason to think that you are somehow less skillful or persistent than those people who overcame their condition quickly?

If you've worked hard on overcoming your condition but are still troubled by it, perhaps there is some significant growth experience to be derived from confronting your difficulty over an extended period of time. For example, many people learn how to let go when they face challenges that don't readily subside. These conditions and situations may be so challenging that they compel us to let go and turn them over to our higher power. To let go and trust in your higher power should not be thought of as foregoing responsibility for your life. Rather, it involves doing all you can to help yourself, while at the same time turning things over to a higher source of assistance.

Creativity gives purpose to life. Creativity doesn't happen only on a canvas. You can inject it into everyday endeavors like cooking or interacting with family members. Creativity comes from *inspiration*, an "influx of spirit." Finding your creative channel and recognizing that you have the ability to produce something that is uniquely your own can give you a sense of ultimate purpose in life. Life can seem incomplete if you don't hone and enjoy your creative gifts, and you may feel more anxiety because you are not expressing your unique talents.

A higher source of support and guidance is always accessible. It's easy to see how accepting or rejecting this idea can factor into your anxiety. Fear and anxiety are based on the perception that you are isolated and vulnerable to the whims of fate. But if you accept that your higher power is always accessible to you, you are no longer alone. Even at those times when you can't turn to others for help, there remains a constant source of support available to you. You can turn to your higher power to receive inspiration and comfort, which can buffer you in rough times. Guidance can come in the form of clear insights and intuitions that provide direction about what you need to do.

Inspiration comes in mundane packages. Inspiration doesn't demand an elaborate setting. Your higher power can manifest itself in day-to-day life. Feelings of awe in the presence of nature, a deep insight that seems to come out of nowhere, synchronicities (uncanny coincidences), and a sudden feeling of support in times of turmoil are some examples of spontaneous spiritual aid and comfort.

Your higher power answers sincere requests. "Ask and you shall receive" may be attributed to Jesus, but it is true regardless of the particular spiritual tradition or orientation you adhere to.

All religions that incorporate prayer hold that prayer will be answered. Perhaps you've had experiences of your prayers being answered. It often seems that the degree of earnestness of your request has something to do with how readily the prayer receives a response. A common example is when you feel overwhelmed with some situation and you almost literally cry out for help to your higher power. In many cases, something about the situation improves or shifts, often within a short time. This doesn't mean that whatever you pray for will come to pass. Prayer can be answered in many ways, and sometimes the answer may not be what you expected. It's not possible to know in advance how a particular prayer will be answered—that is where faith comes in.

What can be trusted is that there will be an answer and that the answer will serve your highest good.

Goals or intentions that come from the deepest level of yourself—from your heart—will be met. A sincerely held intention is a powerful catalyst for positive change. You tend to reach those goals that you believe in and commit to with your whole heart. When the intention is for your own highest good and when it doesn't conflict with anyone else's highest good, it is most likely to become manifest. A deeply held intention shifts and focuses your own consciousness. It also appears to have consequences in the world apart from you. Events in the outer world will actually tend to align with your most deeply held intention.

Each of us is an individualized expression of spirit. There is an aspect of your innermost being that is connected with and an extension of all being. This aspect has been referred to as the self, or *atman* in Eastern philosophy. Many people in the West call it the soul. Transpersonal psychology refers to it as the higher self. The higher self is understood as an individualized or personalized aspect of universal spirit that is at the very center of your being. In short, each of us, at our core, is an individualized expression of the one spirit that exists in all things. Each of us is a drop in the cosmic ocean. It's important to add that your conscious, ego self or personality is not a direct extension of God. Your conscious self (personality) is instead a complex series of concepts, memories, habits, and images that you have created over a lifetime. Who you think you are is something you've learned and created; it is not who you essentially are.

Evil is not a separate force but a misuse of one's creative power. When you're alienated from your innermost being, what you create in your mind as well as in your physical reality is not likely to be beneficial or fulfilling to you and perhaps to others as well. Evil is not an inherent force separate from and against God. (If this were so, God could not be infinite, as something else would exist outside of and independent of God.) It is instead a misuse of our creative power when we make choices that are not in step with our innermost self, our soul. We are not punished by an

angry God for our mistakes; instead, we reap the negative consequences of our own actions that conflict with our higher self
(and thus the universe).

"*Evil*" is a relative term. Eating food that is not healthful
may be out of alignment with your true self but would not usually be called evil. Neither would unintentionally causing an acci-
dent that hurts someone else. Actions labeled evil (intentional
and hurtful crimes, for example) are deliberate and grossly out of
alignment with the perpetrator's innermost being or soul. If, as
has been said, we are all one or joined at the highest level, to
willfully do harm to another is to harm oneself and all of being.
We "should" therefore want to do what is to our highest good—
or what we can intuitively discern to be our highest good—not
because we should do it in any moral sense, but because our
highest good is always what we truly want in our deepest innermost self. In general, when we act out of love or compassion,
we're acting from our innermost being. If there is any ethical
imperative, it is to do what our innermost being or soul truly
wants.

Love is stronger than fear. Pure, unconditional love emanates
from your higher power and is at the very center of your being
and all beings. All fears can be understood as different forms of
separation—separation from others, ourselves, and God. Love is
stronger than fear because it goes deeper. Consciously, love is
the experience of feeling your heart go out toward unity with
someone or something other than yourself. On a deeper level,
love is the ground state or essential foundation of the entire universe. This view is common to both Eastern and Western religions. Love isn't something we either possess or don't possess,
because it literally defines what we are at our core and in our
essence. Fear may go deep, but never as deep as love, because
fear only arises when we feel separate from the ground state that
unifies us with everything else.

Most of the anxiety you experience may be related to specific fears of abandonment, rejection and humiliation, loss of
control, uncertainty, confinement, injury, or death. Fear can take
on any of these forms (and others), based on your conditioning

and past experience. Yet, none of these fears could ever arise if you did not experience separation. The existence of fear always points to a degree of separation of your conscious mind from your innermost being, separation from others, or separation from God.

Death is not an end but a transition. Our essential nature or soul survives physical death. This basic idea is shared by all of the world's religions. They all assert that an individual's soul continues to exist after physical death, although religions differ in their conceptions about the nature of the afterlife.

Does fear of death come up for you or underlie other fears you might have about illness or injury? If so, the idea that your soul is immortal may be comforting to you. You may find it helpful to read about how various faiths view the soul as indestructible. In addition, you may want to read some of the many books and articles written about near-death experiences. The commonality of these experiences from person to person has led to some interesting speculation about life after death.

We hope that the spiritual perspective offered in this chapter will be helpful to you. In considering the ideas offered here, take what fits for you and let go of anything that doesn't. Spirituality is the oldest and most profound pathway to natural healing. Deepening your connection with your higher power can change your life, and may lead to minor or major miracles. At the same time, developing your spiritual life will not eliminate the need to work with the other healing approaches presented in this book. Making time for relaxation and exercise, paying attention to what you eat, thinking realistically, correcting conditions that can aggravate anxiety, utilizing supplements, practicing meditation, and keeping your life simple are all important to help you achieve a calmer, more peaceful way of life.

What spirituality can do is give you inspiration and hope to follow through with your own program for healing yourself. And it can offer you a powerful means for breaking through to your next step forward at those times when you're feeling stuck, discouraged, or confused.

Finding Help from Outside

Though not strictly self-help approaches, there are a number of healing arts practiced by licensed professionals that can be helpful for anxiety. We mention five here that are well known and widely sought after by people dealing with anxiety and other stress-related conditions: massage, acupuncture, chiropractic, homeopathy, and naturopathy. You are likely to derive benefit from any one or all five of these approaches. Weekly treatments of massage, acupuncture, or both can be quite helpful.

Massage

Therapeutic massage is a healing art designed to promote deep relaxation through skillful manipulation of muscles and soft body tissues. Professional massage therapists usually obtain five hundred to a thousand hours of formal training in anatomy, physiology, and various forms of bodywork including Swedish massage, deep-tissue work, reflexology, acupressure, and shiatsu.

Receiving a one-hour massage every week—or even twice a month—can promote deep relaxation by relieving muscle tension that you may have been holding in your body for a long time. Massage can enhance and deepen the benefits of practicing progressive muscle relaxation. Progressive muscle relaxation tends to release acute, superficial tension in the outer muscles of your arms, legs, neck, and torso. Massage, particularly deep-tissue massage, can relieve chronic, long-standing tension held in the deeper muscles of the body. In addition to releasing muscle tension, massage can help cleanse your body of toxic accumulations by promoting lymphatic circulation and mobilizing a sluggish colon.

On a more psychological level, receiving a massage is a wonderful way to nurture yourself if you feel stressed. It can also help you work through any painful feelings or resistance around being touched, increasing your ease with what is an innate need for all human beings.

There are many massage techniques to choose from. *Swedish massage,* developed by Peter Ling in the 1800s, uses kneading, stroking, and shaking to induce the body to relax. This is the most common type of massage. *Deep-tissue massage* involves greater pressure on deeper muscles than Swedish massage and generally focuses on problem areas. *Neuromuscular massage* is a form of deep-tissue massage that works with *trigger points* to release chronically tight muscles. If you'd like to read more about massage, check out *The Massage Book* by George Downing (1972).

Acupuncture

Acupuncture originated as a healing modality in China about three thousand years ago, and it is now practiced throughout the world. As with tai chi, acupuncture holds that health is determined by the free and regular flow of *chi,* the vital or subtle energy that infuses all living things. Chi flows along channels in the body called meridians, each of which is linked to a specific organ. Good health results when the flow of energy is neither restricted nor excessive. If the energy flow is unbalanced in either direction, both physical and mental symptoms of distress or disease may appear. For example, fear is understood to be caused by blocked or excessive energy flow along the kidney meridian. Acupuncture treatments that aim to balance the kidney meridian (and other supporting meridians) can help to relieve fearfulness.

In an acupuncture treatment, the acupuncturist inserts thin needles at specific points in the body. Most people feel only a slight prick or no pain at all from the procedure. Typically the needles are left in place for twenty to thirty minutes, after which it's common to feel very relaxed and rejuvenated. Repeated treatments (twice a week for a few weeks) are often needed to correct an ailment such as migraine headaches, allergies, or back pain. If you wish to utilize acupuncture to help anxiety, weekly or biweekly treatment for several months is advised. Often the acupuncturist will provide herbs in the form of teas or capsules to use at home to enhance the effects of the treatments. Some anxiety sufferers report that they especially benefit from the use of Chinese herbs and continue to rely on them after finishing the acupuncture treatments.

For people who are uncomfortable with the use of needles, *acupressure* may be a viable alternative. Acupressure (and its cousin, *shiatsu*) relies on the same principles as acupuncture; however, energy flow and balance along the meridians is promoted by manual pressure rather than needles. Acupressure is a simple and inexpensive form of energy balance practiced by many massage therapists. You can, in fact, practice acupressure on your own. Michael Gach's 1990 book *Acupressure's Potent Points: A Guide to Self-Care for Common Ailments* provides instructions for self-treatment.

Chiropractic

Most people think of *chiropractic* as a healing art that aims to relieve back pain induced by stress or injury. At a more basic level, though, chiropractic strives to promote health by optimizing the flow of nerve impulses up and down the spine and to other parts of the body. Chiropractic rests on the idea that various stresses on the spine can move individual vertebrae out of alignment, which in turn blocks the flow of nerve impulses between brain and body as well as between the spinal cord and bodily organs. When nerve transmission to a specific organ is reduced or limited, that organ is likely to malfunction, producing symptoms ranging from mild discomfort to illness. Misalignments of the spine may be caused by injury, but most frequently they are caused by stress. Muscles tightened under chronic stress tend to pull the vertebrae out of alignment. Even if the muscle tension is relieved through exercise or massage, the spinal vertebrae may not easily revert to their normal configuration. Thus a chiropractor seeks to identify and correct vertebral misalignments in order to promote optimal nervous system function and thereby functional integrity of the body as a whole.

Chiropractic can be a helpful strategy for relieving chronic tension, whether or not it's accompanied by pain. An occasional visit to a chiropractor may improve your overall experience of well-being. In locating a qualified chiropractor in your area, try to get a referral from a friend or relative. If you prefer not to receive direct manipulations of the spine, there are some chiropractors who practice a nonmanipulative form of adjustment sometimes referred to as *gentle chiropractic.*

Homeopathy

Homeopathy is a system of medicine developed by the German physician Samuel Hahnemann in the late eighteenth century. Homeopathy operates under the principle that any substance that would produce a disease in a healthy person, when given to a sick person with those same disease symptoms, will stimulate a healing response. Homeopathic medicines, called *remedies,* are minute doses of a wide array of natural substances.

Homeopathy may sound very strange if you have only known conventional Western medicine, but it was once quite popular in this country. Then, for a number of reasons—including politics and the emergence of antibiotics—it all but disappeared. There has, however, been a renewal of interest in homeopathy in the past thirty years, coinciding with the rebirth of the natural health movement in this country. Interestingly, homeopathy has always remained a well-utilized form of health care in most of Europe, Latin America, and India.

If you have never seen a homeopath, you are in for a unique experience. The first visit is an interview. Since the remedy you are given is based on the totality of symptoms, many of the questions you will be asked will seem to have nothing to do with your anxiety. To a homeopath, anxiety is just one symptom of a disorder in your total being. You are much more than your anxiety, so to find the right medicine, the homeopath will need to ask many questions about your physical, emotional, and mental health.

Naturopathy

Naturopathy is a method of healing based on the philosophy of *vis medicatrix naturae,* the healing power of nature. The focus of naturopathic medicine is on natural therapies that prevent disease and promote health by stimulating the body's own innate healing abilities. Naturopathic physicians are trained to see the whole person, and so they understand the importance of addressing the interconnectedness of body, mind, and spirit. The training in naturopathic medical schools provides these doctors with thorough grounding in conventional sciences, but they also receive extensive training in areas such as nutrition, botanical medicine, physical medicine, counseling, Chinese medicine, and homeopathy.

A visit to a naturopathic physician may be a very different experience for you. You'll be asked questions about your diet, lifestyle, and emotional health. And instead of leaving with prescription drugs, you'll leave much better educated about how you can assume responsibility for your own health. You will be given specific approaches—perhaps including massage, acupuncture, chiropractic, homeopathy, nutrition, or herbs—that will help you attain your goals.

Comprehensive Wellness Screening

A basic premise of this book is that anxiety difficulties, whatever form they may take, are strongly influenced by your overall level of health and wellness. When your lifestyle supports optimum health, your anxiety will tend to diminish, or, at the very least, be much easier to deal with.

One final approach we recommend to our clients is to undergo a comprehensive wellness screening. This is a battery of tests which you work out with your doctor, usually a holistically oriented physician or a naturopath. Note that most of these tests are not the kind you would receive from a conventional doctor. In fact, they screen for conditions that are often missed by mainstream medicine.

Depending on your particular symptoms, you may complete one or two or perhaps all ten of the assessments listed below. These tests will help you to identify and treat most of the health-related conditions described in this book, and some others we have not discussed. Consult with your holistic physician or naturopath for further information on these tests.

Hair analysis. Screens for mineral deficiencies and heavy metal toxicities.

Glucose tolerance test. Screens for moderate to severe cases of hypoglycemia.

ELISA (enzyme-linked immunosorbent assay) or RAST (radio-allergosorbent test). Comprehensive screening for food allergies

Candida antibodies test (IgG, IgA, IgM). Screens for both intestinal and systemic candidiasis.

Cortisol and DHEA. Measured by blood or saliva tests. Screens for adrenal exhaustion and age-related declines in DHEA.

Comprehensive digestive stool analysis. Screens for parasites, candida, and intestinal dysbiosis. (*Dysbiosis* refers to an unhealthy gut ecology, that is, excessive amounts of unhealthy bacteria such as citrobacter and pseudomonas and insufficient levels of healthy bacteria such as acidophilus and bifidus. Correcting dysbiosis may help many kinds of gastric conditions, including candida and irritable bowel syndrome.)

Complete Thyroid panel (including TSH, T_3, T_4, antithyroglobulin and antithyroperoxidase). Screens for *hyperthyroidism,* which may mimic anxiety disorders, or *hypothyroidism,* which may mimic depression and is often associated with lethargy and fatigue.

Liver enzyme panel. Screens for liver toxicity and general dysfunction.

Kryptopyrroles. Urine test that screens for pyroluria.

Histamine. Blood test that screens for abnormally low or high histamine levels.

Finding Practitioners

Look for holistically oriented MDs or DOs (osteopathic physicians). In certain states, such as Washington, Oregon, Hawaii, Utah, Montana, and Arizona, you may want to work with a naturopath (ND), who has four years of specialized education following three years of premed.

To find a doctor in your area, you can contact:

American College for Advancement of Medicine (ACAM): (949) 583-7666   or   (800) 532-3688;   www.acam.com/doctor search.php.

American Holistic Medical Association (AHMA): (703) 556-9728; www.holisticmedicine.org.

The American Association of Naturopathic Physicians (AANP): (877) 969-2267; www.naturopathic.org.

To find an acupuncturist, you can contact:

National Acupuncture and Oriental Medicine Alliance: (253) 851-6883; www.acull.org.

Further Reading/ Resources

Relaxation

Benson, Herbert. 1975. *The Relaxation Response*. New York: Morrow.

Davis, Martha, Elizabeth Eshelman, and Matthew McKay. 2000. *The Relaxation & Stress Reduction Workbook*. 5th ed. Oakland, Calif.: New Harbinger Publications.

Dr. Emmett Miller offers audio cassettes for relaxation that are soothing and effective. Call Source Cassettes at (800) 52-TAPES or go to www.drmiller.com for a list.

Exercise

Cooper, Robert K. 1989. *Health and Fitness Excellence*. Boston: Houghton Mifflin.

Diet

Balch, James, and Phyllis Balch. 1997. *Prescription for Nutritional Healing*. 2nd ed. Garden City Park, N.Y.: Avery Publishing Group. (A comprehensive reference book.)

Dufty, William. 1974. *Sugar Blues*. New York: Warner Books. (Classic popular book on hypoglycemia.)

Haas, Elson M. 1992. *Staying Healthy with Nutrition*. Berkeley: Celestial Arts. (A very thorough and comprehensive layperson's text on nutrition.)

Robbins, John. 1987. *Diet for a New America*. Walpole, N.H.: Stillpoint Publishing.

Sears, Barry. 1995. *The Zone*. New York: HarperCollins.

Weil, Andrew. 1995. *Natural Health, Natural Medicine*. New York: Houghton Mifflin.

Weil, Andrew. 1995. *Spontaneous Healing*. New York: Fawcett Columbine. (Weil's informative and well-written books have spoken to great numbers of people exploring alternative approaches to health and wellness.)

Thinking Calm

Bourne, Edmund J. 2000. *The Anxiety & Phobia Workbook*. 3rd ed. Oakland, Calif.: New Harbinger Publications.

Bourne, Edmund J., and Lorna Garano. 2003. *Coping with Anxiety*. Oakland, Calif.: New Harbinger Publications.

Helmstetter, Shad. 1982. *What to Say When You Talk to Yourself*. New York: Pocket Books.

McKay, Matthew, Martha Davis, and Patrick Fanning. 1997. *Thoughts and Feelings: The Art of Cognitive Stress Intervention*. 2nd ed. Oakland, Calif.: New Harbinger Publications.

Weekes, Claire. 1978. *Hope and Help for Your Nerves*. New York: Bantam. (A classic in the field that is still helpful today.)

Zeurcher-White, Elke. 1995. *An End to Panic*. Oakland, Calif.: New Harbinger Publications.

Conditions That Can Affect Anxiety

(The books by Larson and Ross are especially helpful for an in-depth discussion of various conditions that can affect anxiety and mood disorder.)

Bender, Stephanie. 1989. *PMS: Questions and Answers*. Los Angeles: Sloan.

Crook, William. 1989. *The Yeast Connection*. 3rd ed. Jackson, Tenn.: Professional Books.

Larson, Joan Mathews. 1999. *Depression Free, Naturally*. New York: Ballantine.

Ross, Julia. 2002. *The Mood Cure*. New York: Penguin Books.

Rosenthal, Norman. 1993. *Winter Blues: Seasonal Affective Disorder and How to Overcome It*. New York: Guilford Press.

Wilson, James L. 2001. *Adrenal Fatigue*. Petaluma, Calif.: Smart Publications. (A comprehensive book on adrenal exhaustion.)

Information about companies that manufacture light therapy devices is available from the National Organization for Seasonal Affective Disorder (NOSAD), P.O. Box 40133, Washington DC 20016. NOSAD offers a number of resources including basic information, a bibliography, and a support network of people across the country you can call.

Supplements

Bloomfield, Harold. 1998. *Healing Anxiety with Herbs*. New York: HarperCollins.

Bloomfield, Harold, Mikael Nordfors, and Peter McWilliams. 1996. *Hypericum & Depression*. Santa Monica, Calif.: Prelude Press.

Brown, Richard. 1999. *Stop Depression Now*. New York: Putnam. (A comprehensive book on SAM-e.)

Cass, Hyla, and Terrence McNally. 1998. *Kava: Nature's Answer to Stress, Anxiety, and Insomnia*. Rocklin, Calif.: Prima Health.

Davidson, Jonathan, and Kathryn M. Connor. 2000. *Herbs for the Mind*. New York: Guilford Press.

Larson, Joan Mathews. 1999. *Depression Free, Naturally*. New York: Ballantine.

Ley, Beth M. 1996. *DHEA: Unlocking the Secrets to the Fountain of Youth*. Newport Beach, Calif.: BML Publications.

Mindell, Earl. 1979. *Vitamin Bible*. New York: Warner Books.

Mindell, Earl. 1992. *Herb Bible*. New York: Fireside Books.

Ross, Julia. 2002. *The Mood Cure*. New York: Penguin Books.

Slagle, Priscilla. 1987. *The Way Up from Down*. New York: Random House.

Tierra, Michael. 1990. *The Way of Herbs*. New York: Pocket Books.

Weil, Andrew. 1995. *Natural Health, Natural Medicine*. New York: Houghton Mifflin.

Meditation

Goldstein, Joseph, and Jack Kornfield. 1987. *Seeking the Heart of Wisdom: The Path of Insight Meditation*. Boston: Shambhala.

Harp, David. 1996. *The Three-Minute Meditator*. 3rd ed. Oakland, Calif.: New Harbinger Publications.

Kabat-Zinn, Jon. 1990. *Full Catastrophe Living*. New York: Delta.

Kabat-Zinn, Jon. 1994. *Wherever You Go, There You Are*. New York: Hyperion.

Kornfield, Jack. 1993. *A Path with Heart*. New York: Bantam.

LeShan, Lawrence. 1974. *How to Meditate*. New York: Bantam.

Levine, Stephen. 1989. *A Gradual Awakening*. New York: Anchor.

Mindful Exercise

Basic Yoga Workout for Dummies. 2001. Anchor Bay Entertainment. VHS and DVD.

Cohen, Ken. 1996. *Qi gong: Traditional Chinese Exercises for Healing Body, Mind, and Spirit*. Sounds True Video. VHS.

Eight Simple Qi gong Exercises for Health. 2003. YMA Publication Center. VHS.

Hessel, Jillian. 2003. *Pilates for Beginners.* Living Arts. VHS and DVD.

Hittleman, Richard. 1985. *Yoga for Health.* New York: Ballantine.

Iyengar, B. K. 1995. *Light on Yoga.* New York: Schocken Books.

Lam, Paul. 2001. *Tai Chi—The 24 Forms.* VHS and DVD.

McFarland, Stewart, and Mew Mong Tan. 1997. *Complete Book of T'ai Chi.* New York: DK Publishing.

Pierce, Margaret, and Martin Pierce. 1996. *Yoga for Life.* Portland, Oreg.: Rudra Press.

Pilates Beginning Mat Workout. 2000. Living Arts. VHS and DVD.

Pilates for Dummies. 2001. Anchor Bay Entertainment. DVD.

Qi gong for Healing. 2003. Living Arts. VHS.

Sacred Yoga Practice—Vinyasa Flow. 2003. Goldhill Home Media I. VHS and DVD.

Shou-yu Liang and Wen-ching Wu. 1996. *Qi gong Empowerment: A Guide to Medical, Taoist, Buddhist Wushus Energy Cultivation.* East Providence, R.I.: Way of Dragon Press.

Tai Chi—Energy Training for Mind & Body, vols. 1 and 2. 2003. Golden Pictures. DVD.

Yoga Zone—Yoga Basics 5 Pack. 2002. Koch Vision Entertainment. VHS.

Keep It Simple

Eisenson, Marc, Gerri Detweiler, and Nancy Castleman. 2001. *Stop Junk Mail Forever.* Elizaville, N.Y.: Good Advice Press.

Elgin, Duane. 1993. *Voluntary Simplicity.* New York: William Morrow.

Fanning, Patrick, and Heather Garnos Mitchener. 2001. *The 50 Best Ways to Simplify Your Life.* Oakland, Calif.: New Harbinger Publications.

Mundis, Jerold. 1990. *How to Get Out of Debt, Stay Out of Debt, and Live Prosperously.* New York: Bantam.

St. James, Elaine. 1994. *Simplify Your Life.* New York: Hyperion.

Spirituality

Borysenko, Joan. 1993. *Fire in the Soul*. New York: Warner Books.

Bunick, Nick. 1998. *In God's Truth*. Charlottesville, Va.: Hampton Roads Publishing.

Caddy, Eileen. 1979. *The Dawn of Change*. Forres, Scotland: Findhorn Publications.

Chopra, Deepak. 1994. *The Seven Spiritual Laws of Success*. San Rafael, Calif.: New World Library.

Dossey, Larry. 1989. *Recovering the Soul: A Scientific and Spiritual Search*. New York: Bantam.

Harmon, Willis. 1988. *Global Mind Change*. New York: Warner Books.

Moody, Raymond. 1976. *Life After Life*. New York: Bantam.

Norwood, Robin. 1994. *Why Me, Why This, Why Now*. New York: Carol Southern Books.

Peck, Scott. 1978. *The Road Less Traveled*. New York: Simon & Schuster.

Peck, Scott. 1993. *Further Along the Road Less Traveled*. New York: Simon & Schuster.

Redfield, James. 1993. *The Celestine Prophecy*. New York: Warner Books.

Ring, Kenneth. 1985. *Heading toward Omega*. New York: William Morrow.

Rodegast, Pat. 1985. *Emmanuel's Book*. New York: Bantam.

Rodegast, Pat. 1989. *Emmanuel's Book, II*. New York: Bantam.

Talbot, Michael. 1992. *The Holographic Universe*. New York: HarperCollins.

Virtue, Doreen. 1998. *Divine Guidance*. New York: Warner Books.

Walsch, Neale. 1996. *Conversations with God (Book I)*. New York: Putnam.

Williamson, Marianne. 1994. *Illuminata*. New York: Random House.

Zukav, Gary. 1990. *The Seat of the Soul*. New York: Fireside Books.

Chapter References

Chapter 1

Benson, Herbert. 1975. *The Relaxation Response.* New York: Bantam Books.

Jacobson, Edmond. 1974. *Progressive Relaxation.* Midway Reprint. Chicago: University of Chicago Press.

Chapter 3

Sears, Barry. 1995. *The Zone.* New York: HarperCollins.

Chapter 4

Weekes, Claire. 1978. *Hope and Help for Your Nerves.* New York: Bantam Books.

Chapter 5

Larson, Joan Mathews. 1999. *Depression Free, Naturally*. New York: Ballantine.

Pfeiffer, Carl. 1975. *Mental and Elemental Nutrients: A Physical Guide to Nutrition and Health Care*. New Canaan, Conn.: Keats Publishing.

Rosenthal, Norman. 1993. *Winter Blues: Seasonal Affective Disorder and How to Overcome It*. New York: Guilford Press.

Seyle, Hans. 1984. *The Stress of Life*. New York: McGraw-Hill.

Chapter 6

Bloomfield, Harold, Mikael Nordfors, and Peter McWilliams. 1996. *Hypericum & Depression*. Santa Monica, Calif.: Prelude Press.

Brown, Richard. 1999. *Stop Depression Now*. New York: Putnam.

Cass, Hyla, and Terrence McNally. 1998. *Kava: Nature's Answer to Stress, Anxiety, and Insomnia*. Rocklin, Calif.: Prima Health.

Davidson, Jonathan, and Kathryn M. Connor. 2000. *Herbs for the Mind*. New York: Guilford Press.

Dragull, Klaus, Wesley Y. Yoshida, and Chung-shih Tang. 2003. Piperidine alkaloids from *Piper methysticum*. *Phytochemistry* 63(2):193–98.

Chapter 7

Kabat-Zinn, Jon. 1990. *Full Catastrophe Living*. New York: Delta.

———. 1994. *Wherever You Go, There You Are*. New York: Hyperion.

Chapter 8

Goldberg, Burton. 1993. *Alternative Therapies*. Fife, Wash.: Future Medicine Publishing, Inc.

Chapter 9

Elgin, Duane. 1993. *Voluntary Simplicity*. New York: William Morrow.

Fanning, Patrick, and Heather Garnos Mitchener. 2001. *The 50 Best Ways to Simplify Your Life*. Oakland, Calif.: New Harbinger Publications.

Edmund J. Bourne, Ph.D., has specialized in the treatment of anxiety disorders and related problems for two decades. For many years, he was director of the Anxiety Treatment Center in San Jose and Santa Rosa, CA. His best-selling anxiety workbooks, which have helped hundreds of thousands of readers throughout the world, include *The Anxiety and Phobia Workbook*, *Beyond Anxiety and Phobia*, and *Coping with Anxiety*. He lives and practices in Hawaii and California.

Arlen Brownstein, MS, ND, is a naturopathic physician. She earned her ND from Bastyr University in Seattle, WA. After completing her undergraduate degree at the University of California, Berkeley, she earned a master's degree in nutrition from the University of Connecticut in Storrs, CT. She is the author of *Rosacea: Your Self-Help Guide*.

Lorna Garano is a freelance writer and editor living in Oakland, CA.

Individual phone consultations are available with Dr. Bourne. Comprehensive treatment programs and retreats utilizing a natural approach are also available in Hawaii and California. For further information, please contact (808) 334-1847.

Some Other New Harbinger Titles

Surviving Your Borderline Parent, Item 3287 $14.95

When Anger Hurts, second edition, Item 3449 $16.95

Calming Your Anxious Mind, Item 3384 $12.95

Ending the Depression Cycle, Item 3333 $17.95

Your Surviving Spirit, Item 3570 $18.95

Coping with Anxiety, Item 3201 $10.95

The Agoraphobia Workbook, Item 3236 $19.95

Loving the Self-Absorbed, Item 3546 $14.95

Transforming Anger, Item 352X $10.95

Don't Let Your Emotions Run Your Life, Item 3090 $17.95

Why Can't I Ever Be Good Enough, Item 3147 $13.95

Your Depression Map, Item 3007 $19.95

Successful Problem Solving, Item 3023 $17.95

Working with the Self-Absorbed, Item 2922 $14.95

The Procrastination Workbook, Item 2957 $17.95

Coping with Uncertainty, Item 2965 $11.95

The BDD Workbook, Item 2930 $18.95

You, Your Relationship, and Your ADD, Item 299X $17.95

The Stop Walking on Eggshells Workbook, Item 2760 $18.95

Conquer Your Critical Inner Voice, Item 2876 $15.95

The PTSD Workbook, Item 2825 $17.95

Hypnotize Yourself Out of Pain Now!, Item 2809 $14.95

The Depression Workbook, 2nd edition, Item 268X $19.95

Beating the Senior Blues, Item 2728 $17.95

Call **toll free, 1-800-748-6273,** or log on to our online bookstore at **www.newharbinger.com** to order. Have your Visa or Mastercard number ready. Or send a check for the titles you want to New Harbinger Publications, Inc., 5674 Shattuck Ave., Oakland, CA 94609. Include $4.50 for the first book and 75¢ for each additional book, to cover shipping and handling. (California residents please include appropriate sales tax.) Allow two to five weeks for delivery.

Prices subject to change without notice.